What to Pray
When You Are Expecting

Hopes, Prayers, and Dreams During Pregnancy—
for Mom and the Whole Family

Joyce Penner

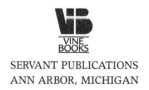

VINE
BOOKS

SERVANT PUBLICATIONS
ANN ARBOR, MICHIGAN

Vine Books is an imprint of Servant Publications especially designed to serve evangelical Christians.

Scripture verses marked NASB are from the New American Standard Bible, © The Lockman Foundation 1960, 1962, 1963, 1968, 1971, 1972, 1973, 1975, 1977. Scripture quotations marked NLT are taken from the *Holy Bible,* New Living Translation, © 1996. Used by permission of Tyndale House Publishers, Inc., Wheaton, Illinois 60189. All rights reserved. Scripture quotations from THE MESSAGE, © Eugene H. Peterson 1993, 1994, 1995. Used by permission of NavPress Publishing Group.

Published by Servant Publications
P.O. Box 8617
Ann Arbor, Michigan 48107

Cover design: Left Coast Design, Inc. Portland, Oregon
Cover photograph: © Rob Lewine / The Stock Market

00 01 02 03 10 9 8 7 6 5 4 3 2 1

Printed in the United States of America
ISBN 1-56955-135-9

LIBRARY OF CONGRESS CATALOGING-IN-PUBLICATION DATA

Penner, Joyce.
    What to pray when you are expecting : hopes, prayers, and dreams during pregnancy—for mom and the whole family / Joyce Penner.
      p.   cm.
    Includes bibliographical references.
    ISBN 1-56955-135-9 (alk. paper)
    1. Pregnant women—Religious life. 2. Pregnancy—Religious aspects—Christianity. I. Title.
    BV4529.18.P46   2000
    242'.6431—dc21   00-026719

Contents

Dedication

To my children and grandchildren:
John, Julene, and Matthew;
Gregory, Carrie, Kevin, and Drew;
Kristine and her future husband;
and all future grandchildren.
In these pages I express many of my passions for life
that I hope I have demonstrated
as your mother and grandmother.

Acknowledgments

Without my family, this book would not be possible. My husband Cliff was his usual servant helper self. My daughters were incredible! A very special thank you to Julene, who spent hours not only editing but also evaluating the content from the perspective of a child and adolescent psychologist and the mother of a one-year-old. A thank you to Carrie, educational consultant and pregnant mother of a two-year-old, whose vulnerable input positively guided the tone with which I communicated my passions. And thank you to Kristine for her editing and especially her technical input and corrections from her perspective as a human biologist.

Thank you to my official editors, Kathryn Deering and Sandy Judd, for patience, expertise, and continued affirmation and encouragement. And finally, a big thank you to our assistant, Kathy Killebrew, for always being willing to be there to bail me out of computer frustrations and deadline pressures.

Preface

Prayer, pregnancy, and parenting are intricately interwoven in who I am as a person. Prayer and parenting are as fundamental to me as eating and sleeping. During my pregnancies, prayer and faith in God were indispensable. This was especially true of my second pregnancy.

It was early summer 1969. I was sitting at a luncheon. My husband, Cliff, was already at the event when I arrived after my doctor's appointment for my twelfth-week pregnancy checkup. I can still picture myself at the end of the table, hearing the buzzing of voices but taking in no words. People were all around me, but I saw no one. I was overwhelmed by emotion but could feel nothing. God seemed far away. I was totally numb.

My obstetrician had just informed me that my blood titer indicated that the slight fever and rash I had experienced two weeks before had been German measles. As warmly as he could, he had told me that I had only a 10 percent chance of bringing home a normal baby. Severe deformities were a most likely consequence. As a believer himself, he had had difficulty making the suggestion that Cliff and I consider abortion, but as a physician in an era without ultrasound technology he believed he needed to present that option.

The months that followed became a time of deepening prayer and faith, accompanied by a blur of emotions. My contractions started six weeks before my January 6 due date, and I was given medication to slow down the process until December 18, when my physician determined it would be best to induce me. A private room was set up for me and the baby, since the baby could not be taken into the nursery for fear of contaminating other newborns with the virus it would be carrying. Pediatric neonatal specialists were on hand to await the birth.

Forty-five minutes after the medication to induce my labor was started, I delivered the most perfect, beautiful baby boy, Gregory Boyd Penner! I shook for an hour as Cliff and I, with tears of joy streaming down our faces, watched the nurses and doctors examine our baby. Every one of his bodily systems was normal. How grateful we were for the faith that had given us the courage not to abort, and the hope, despite fears, that had strengthened us throughout the pregnancy.

Prayer is essential to parenting, and of course, parenting begins with pregnancy. Since you have purchased this book or received it as a gift, perhaps you (or your wife) are expecting or thinking of having a child. Wonderful! Now is the time to start praying for that anticipated child!

Every person has different experiences with prayer. My prayer life began with two recited prayers. The first I learned to say with my mother at bedtime after she read me a Bible story. It is a familiar one:

> Now I lay me down to sleep,
> I pray thee, Lord, my soul to keep.
> If I should die before I wake,
> I pray thee, Lord, my soul to take. Amen.

The second prayer my three brothers, my sister, and I took turns reciting before meals.

God is great, God is good,
And we thank Him for this food. Amen.

Beyond such simple rituals, prayer became personal for me at age six. At the same time, it became self-consciously private and thoughtfully serious.

I was attending Daily Vacation Bible School, a summer children's program at a local Mennonite church in our little rural community in southwestern Minnesota. My age group met in the basement of that church in a small cubicle—a portion of a larger room separated by a curtain on a rod. I don't remember much about the lesson that day, but I can still picture myself walking up the stairs out of that basement room with a sense of awe that I was different. I had asked to stay after class and had knelt and prayed with my teacher to ask Jesus to come into my life and be my Lord and Savior.

I came home, greeted my mother in the kitchen, and went directly to the bathroom upstairs to be alone and pray. I did not share my experience with anyone; it was too sacred to be made known.

Certainly as sacred but hardly as private are pregnancy and parenthood. They are responsibilities I took as seriously as my communication with God. I studied prenatal nutrition and exercise, child development, developmental psychology, and everything I could find in the Bible on parenting—both direct and indirect teachings—and I read the parenting books available at that time. My husband and I took every class we could find on the subject. I approached pregnancy, labor, delivery, and parenting with informed anticipation.

Parenting has been the most rewarding job I have ever assumed. What a joy it is to be a mom and grandma! Because of the passion I feel for motherhood, God has placed in my life various mothers whom I have mentored. I began mentoring other new moms more than twenty years ago, long before mentoring was a common concept. The oldest child of these treasured friends is now in her midtwenties.

Unfortunately, I didn't prepare myself as thoroughly for grandmothering. I didn't even realize preparation was needed. I assumed that my comfort in parenting and helping others parent would make me equally natural at grandmothering. I was taken by surprise and had to learn after the fact. Fortunately, our children have been gracious in teaching me how they need me to grandmother their children.

You may be coming to parenting with similar assumptions. Beware! Each of life's transitions requires adjustment. Pregnancy and parenting are complex transformations and bring an intense range of emotions. Even though the first pregnancy elicits the most change and anticipation of the unknown, the making of each new child is a unique event.

Preparation, faith, and information will empower you to embrace this exciting life adventure with courage and joy. With knowledge and trust in God, you will be able to safely navigate the perplexing, ever-changing road of pregnancy and parenting. Yet the inexhaustible supply of information and tips for parenting today can be overwhelming for the eager couple.

This book is intended as a companion to give you confidence through the nine months of your pregnancy and to provide you with a framework for approaching the information you will encounter. First we'll take a deeper look at prayer, pregnancy, and parenting. Then we'll walk through the month-by-month milestones: the growth of the developing baby, the changes in and needs of the mother's body, and the necessary adjustments of the couple and family. You will be challenged with a monthly decision regarding pregnancy and parenting and directed to specific resources to help you in your decision-making process. You will be encouraged to think about opposing views related to those decisions, and be directed in making the best use of the information and resources available. Prayers related to each decision and month's events will be a stimulus to your own prayer life. Suggestions for you to record your prayer requests and answers will provide opportunities to connect all that is happening physically with your spirituality.

I hope you will trust and follow the footsteps of the One who will walk with you on every path of this child-producing and child rearing journey. May the words that I share in these pages be stepping stones of wisdom, faith, peace, and joy that direct you along the first nine-month path of this lifelong adventure.

> God, the one and only—
> ... Everything I hope for comes from him,
> ... He's solid rock under my feet,
> ... An impregnable castle:
> I'm set for life.
>
> PSALM 62:6-7, THE MESSAGE

Don't fret or worry. Instead of worrying, pray. Let petitions and praises shape your worries into prayers, letting God know your concerns. Before you know it, a sense of God's wholeness, everything coming together for good, will come and settle you down. It's wonderful what happens when Christ displaces worry at the center of your life.

PHILIPPIANS 4:6-7, THE MESSAGE

On Prayer

Prayer changes us. It touches us at the very center of our lives. Through prayer we draw closer to God and allow Him to draw closer to us. It is through prayer that we accept the realization that we have access to God—to His holiness and His power. When we worry, we are trying to control that which is not in our control. Even the best of us worry about pregnancy and raising children. What a comfort when we are able to enlist God's power through prayer and allow Christ to displace our worries with trust in the knowledge that He is in control.

In the sixth chapter of Matthew, Jesus is talking to His followers. His words teach us to release our concerns for food and clothing and our future to God and allow Him to care for us. He ends that passage with these thoughts:

Give your entire attention to what God is doing right now, and don't get worked up about what may or may not happen tomorrow. God will help you deal with whatever hard things come up when the time comes.

MATTHEW 6:34, THE MESSAGE

Rest assured that "hard things" will indeed come up as you live out the role of parents. The awesome responsibility of parenting brings most of us to God in prayer. We don't know what the future holds for these innocent, totally dependent little lives. Whatever our tradition or practice has been, there is a new awareness of our inadequacy and our dependence on God's intimate involvement in our lives.

Even though I was raised in a home of deep Christian faith, personal prayer was not overtly modeled for me. Verbally expressed prayers were memorized recitations. Yet, I somehow knew my mother and father were in daily interaction with God. My mom had her Bible beside her bed with a devotional guidebook. Both were used and marked. My dad would spend long private periods with his Bible.

I learned to pray publicly in our Mennonite church of sixty-five members, but my doing so disturbed my Mennonite grandfather deeply. Praying out loud was a public show. He and some of our Mennonite forefathers took most seriously and very literally the Matthew 6 passage in which Jesus teaches us to pray in private and with simplicity.

And when you pray, you are not to be as the hypocrites; for they love to stand and pray in the synagogues and on the street corners, in order to be seen by men. Truly I say to you, they have their reward in full. But you, when you pray, go into your inner room, and when you have shut your door, pray to your Father....

MATTHEW 6:5-6, NASB

You may have learned to pray through the rituals of coming into the presence of God practiced in the Roman Catholic Church. You may have had intense emotional prayer times as part of a charismatic movement, where you experienced divine intervention through the presence of the Holy Spirit and your language and your body expressed the cries of your heart. You may have been taught traditional Jewish blessings. You may be one who comes to God only in desperation at times of crises.

Whatever your past experience with prayer, this stage of life may elicit a new longing for intimacy with God. As you look for growth in your prayer life, learn from those around you. Join a church or group with whom you can worship. Attend to God's prompting as you pray.

I currently serve on the Ministry Council of Lake Avenue Church in Pasadena, California. We, as a council, seek God not only for wisdom and guidance in governing the body of Christ's followers who have entrusted themselves to us as their leaders, but also for spiritual growth and renewal. My charismatic peer on the council is a wonderful contrast and model to me of expressing her interaction with God with her whole being. I at times feel very limited in my freedom to audibly approach God with my true praise and deep concerns in the presence of others. I find myself so controlled by my grandfather's fear of public display that my words become the performance Matthew 6 warns against. But as I have learned to share my prayers aloud within this community of believers, I have grown deeply.

Prayer has been continuous in and vital to my life. It is a moment-by-moment trust and interaction with God that has given me an inner strength and a deep peace ever since I was six years old. I have had to learn to bring that meaningful private interaction with God into my relationships with others. For even as the Scriptures teach that we are not to pray for the purpose of public attention and display, they also inform us that where two or three are gathered in prayer, God is there, hearing and caring. We are encouraged to pray with others.

Why Are We to Pray?

Prayer helps us persist and not give up; it instills hope.
Prayer increases our faith.
Prayer helps us focus our perspective on God.
Prayer clarifies our needs, desires, and requests.
Prayer maintains and strengthens our relationship with God.
Prayer is a path to power, an answer to our helplessness.
Prayer helps us surrender our ways to God's desires for us.
Prayer does not always bring us our wants, but it leads us to more clearly understand God's love and care for us, His children.

With all prayer and petition pray at all times in the Spirit.

EPHESIANS 6:18a, NASB

God's Word is an indispensable weapon. In the same way, prayer is essential in this ongoing warfare. Pray hard and long.

EPHESIANS 6:17-18, THE MESSAGE

How Are We to Pray?

We are to pray with simplicity.
We are to pray with submission to God's will.
We are to pray expectantly.
We are to pray with our focus on God, not ourselves.
We are to pray with persistence.

When Jesus went up on the mountain to teach His disciples, He taught them lessons for life (the Beatitudes), explained their purpose in the world, and gave them guidelines for personal relationships and emotional well-being. He also taught them how to pray (see Matthew 6). He encouraged them not to draw attention to themselves or their good deeds, and not to just repeat words that soon would become meaningless, but rather to recognize that our Father knows what we need even before we ask Him. He said, "Pray, then, in this way":

Our Father, who art in heaven, hallowed be Thy name, Thy kingdom come. Thy will be done, on earth as it is in heaven. Give us this day our daily bread. And forgive us our debts, as we also have forgiven our debtors. And do not lead us into temptation, but deliver us from evil. For Thine is the kingdom, and the power, and the glory, forever, Amen.

MATTHEW 6:9-13, NASB

The Lord's Prayer, or the Our Father, is the ecumenical Christian prayer. It is a simple, basic prayer that honors God, recognizes His power, assumes hope, places the person offering the prayer in the province of God's will, and then brings to Him our human needs for food, forgiveness, and protection from wrongdoing.

In addition to the model of the Lord's Prayer, I draw on others' teachings. The methods of prayer I have gleaned from C.S. Lewis' book *Letters to Malcolm: Chiefly on Prayer*[1] have been key to my prayer life. He talks about *prayer without words,* or praying with mental images, as the most wonderful experience of communicating with God, but cautions that this form of prayer carries the risk of "becoming merely [an] imaginative or emotional act."

Lewis sees *using one's own words* as the staple of prayer, but he cautions against letting our homemade prayers harden into formulas of unavoidable repetition. Prayers of our own devising flow from deep within.

"A ready-made form can't serve for ... intercourse with God any more than it could serve for" intercourse with another person. *Ready-made prayers,* however, serve several functions: they keep us in touch with sound doctrine, they remind us of what we ought to ask, and they provide a ceremonial element.

I find I incorporate all three of Lewis' prayer methods in my prayer times. When I was bedridden with rheumatic fever as a junior in high school, the prayers of my heart often flowed from within me as mental images rather than words. These were moments of passionate closeness with God. To this day, I continually talk with God, sometimes in words and sometimes by picturing Him wrapping His arms around a particular person or situation.

In the morning, the Lord's Prayer is the ready-made model I use to guide my requests and keep me focused on God rather than myself. I began using this format after my father was found dead of a massive heart attack just one year after my mother's sudden death. I was too taken by grief to be able to sense God's presence or gain access to Him. Such a sense of isolation from God is common when we are stressed, over-whelmed, or depressed. I now use the Lord's Prayer daily, filling in my own words and mental images.

"Our Father, who art in heaven" helps me to put God first. For me it is not difficult to address God as a loving, caring, and providing Father because my earthly father filled that role. If you did not grow up with a perception of your own father as someone who cares for you and wants the best for you, you may have more difficulty experiencing God as a patient, tender Father.

"Hallowed be Thy name" conjures within me an attitude of worship, in which I can honor God's holiness and surrender to Him every compartment of my life. I use my own words to express my highest regard for His willingness to meet me through Jesus Christ, and I picture myself open and vulnerable before Him.

"Thy kingdom come. Thy will be done, on earth as it is in heaven" becomes specific and personal for the concerns and issues of each day. I picture and use my own words to bring to God my husband, each of our children and grandchildren, extended family members, my prayer partners and their families, friends, the pastors and leadership of our church, world and political issues, and those I care for in my profession and ministries. I plead for His will and power to be put into action to give strength to those in need, so that we might experience His kingdom—His ways—here on earth in our everyday lives.

"Give us this day our daily bread" is usually praise for how generously we have been blessed, but also a prayer for wise use of our resources and generosity toward those in need. There are times when I have needed to ask for provisions. I also focus on bodily needs and praises for health.

"And forgive us our debts, as we also have forgiven our

debtors" is an important reminder to me that I am to treat others as God has so generously treated me. When the children were young, I thought often of how I would want God to acknowledge me when I wasn't at my best. I tried to respond to my needy little ones with that same open heart.

"And do not lead us into temptation, but deliver us from evil" is a constant prayer.

When Are We to Pray?

We are to pray without ceasing. As a parent, you will likely find, as I have, and as C.S. Lewis writes to his friend Malcolm: "My own plan, when hard pressed, is to seize any time, and place, however unsuitable, in preference to the last waking moment. On a day of traveling ... I'd rather pray sitting in a crowded train [for me, an airplane or car] than put it off till midnight when one reaches a hotel bedroom with aching head and dry throat and one's mind partly in a stupor and partly in a whirl."[2]

If you are a new mother, you might pray while walking, breastfeeding, changing, rocking, or patting the baby. You may find yourself in prayer while lying in bed listening to see if your little one has fallen asleep or still needs you to help her settle down. Just this week, I had a mother with her baby in my office expressing deep concern over her current lack of spirituality. She had been accustomed to taking an hour a day to read the Bible and pray. She was now condemning herself for not keeping that routine since the baby arrived. I suspect that God is blessing her for the time she is devoting to honoring Him by giving herself and her time to her young child, rather than judging her.

Having a baby will change every one of your patterns of daily living, including prayer. Adapting disciplines of pre-baby life to the new demands on your time can be a challenge. Allow yourself much grace.

Prayers and Children

The people brought children to Jesus, hoping he might touch them. The disciples shooed them off. But Jesus was irate and let them know it: "Don't push these children away. Don't ever get between them and me. These children are at the very center of life in the kingdom." ... Then, gathering the children up in his arms, he laid his hands of blessing on them.

MARK 10:13-16, THE MESSAGE

Jesus taught his followers an important lesson about the value of bringing our children to Him. We can bring our children to God in prayer before they have even been conceived. God made that message clear in these words to the prophet Jeremiah:

Before I formed you in the womb I knew you,
And before you were born I consecrated you.

JEREMIAH 1:5a, NASB

For many of us, our first petition to God for our children was a desire to conceive. We so often take gifts like conception for granted. We assume we will become pregnant. Yet infertility is a devastation to many couples. On the other hand, unexpected pregnancies or those being experienced by women alone can require huge adjustments. Whether your pregnancy was intended or not, in Scripture pregnancy is viewed as a blessing.

> From the God of your father who helps you,
> And by the Almighty who blesses you
> With blessings of heaven above,
> Blessings of the deep that lies beneath,
> Blessings of the breasts and of the womb.
>
> GENESIS 49:25, NASB

During pregnancy, prayers for our children tend to focus on healthy development and safety throughout the pregnancy and delivery. In some ways, our prayers are similar after our children are born.

Through prayer we bring our children to God and ask Him to care for them, protect them, and meet their needs. Even as in the Old Testatment Scriptures Samuel's mother, Hannah, recognized her son as a gift from God, so should we also thank God for the miracle of our children and dedicate them to Him.

> And she said, "Oh my lord! As your soul lives, my lord, I am the woman who stood here beside you, praying to the Lord. For this boy I prayed, and the Lord has given me my petition which I asked of Him. So I have also dedicated him to the Lord, as long as he lives he is dedicated to the Lord.
>
> 1 SAMUEL 1:26-28, NASB

Children are not ours to possess, whether born to us or adopted by us. Rather, they are an entrustment from God. It is our responsibility to nurture each one physically, emotionally, and spiritually. That responsibility starts the moment we prepare to conceive. As mothers-to-be we take care of our bodies. Fathers-to-be also need to prepare their bodies for conception, to increase the number, health, and even the vigor of their sperm. In addition to the physical preparation, however, spiritual preparation is also essential. Praying for both the physical and spiritual development of our child prepares us emotionally for the transition into parenthood.

After a discussion of the roles and responsibilities of parenting, I will look at each month of development, focusing on specific prayers and Scriptures for each month. Pregnancy is the time to make a commitment to be a prayer ally for your child. Both you and your child will benefit.

Don't you see that children are God's best gift?
    the fruit of the womb his generous legacy?
Like a warrior's fistful of arrows
    are the children of a vigorous youth.
Oh, how blessed are you parents,
    with your quivers full of children!

PSALM 127: 4-5, THE MESSAGE

On Pregnancy

Pregnancy changes our lives forever. For most, it is a welcome and exciting change. Pregnancy is one of the happiest times in many young couples' lives. If you can, embrace this life transition by becoming informed and preparing for the wonderful and challenging events that are just beginning. The formation of a baby in the mother's womb is portrayed in the Scriptures as an awesome mystery attributed to God's care and intervention.

Whether planned or unplanned, whether the timing is perfect or couldn't be worse, pregnancy is a crisis. Coping with change, even good change, stirs up ambivalence and stress.

Much like pregnancy, the marriage of one's child engenders emotions impossible to identify and label. I remember sitting on a pew in the back of the church before our oldest daughter's wedding. One of Julene's bridesmaids, noticing my pensive gaze, sat down beside me. She had gotten married a few months before. She put into words my feelings, which until she verbalized them had been unknown to me. I can't recall exactly what she said, but it was something about how many emotions I must be experiencing, anticipating the marriage of my oldest daughter. How true! That is the nature of change: it pulls us in opposing directions. We love it, yet it also frightens us. We so want our children to find joy and contentment. Yet we fear the multitude of potential obstacles they will face in achieving their dreams.

Although some women keep an even disposition throughout pregnancy, most struggle with intense, fluctuating feelings. You may be happy and excited one moment, then find yourself irritable, worried, or weepy the next. Your feelings may surprise you. It is important that you recognize that your changing emotions are normal. If you closely monitor what you are feeling and ask for the support you need from your husband and family, you and they will not be overwhelmed by your moods.

As husband and wife or as a single mom-to-be, your reaction to your pregnancy depends so much on your life situation and your circumstances. Your financial status, your marital relationship, your living conditions, your health, the other demands on your time and energy, and your community or family support will factor into your feelings.

The months until the baby arrives will require careful planning, adjustments, and some hard work. The more information you and your family have, the better you will be able to anticipate and adapt to the changes pregnancy and parenting demand.

There are many advantages to having a baby in this day and age. If you have Internet access or any of the many books on pregnancy, you can be informed about every change that is happening in your body and the baby's growth and development. You can learn what to take into your body and what to avoid, how to exercise, what to do if you experience certain symptoms, and how to prepare for labor and delivery. Your interaction with your physician need not be dependent on what he or she shares with you. You will probably come to appointments with questions about what you already have read or seen. Hopefully your doctor will welcome your exposure to this wealth of data.

Even though it is natural to have fears, it is so much safer to have a baby today than it was even twenty or thirty years ago. All aspects of prenatal care and testing, monitoring of the mother and her baby in labor, and outcomes for high risk babies and mothers have dramatically improved. The amount of information available and the technological advances in medicine in recent decades can dispel those concerns and make your pregnancy a richly rewarding time that you will remember with fondness.

Care for Yourself

Get Yourself Healthy Before You Get Yourself a Baby

Our friend and colleague Dr. Neil Clark Warren, in his book *Finding the Love of Your Life*, recommends that individuals get themselves healthy before they get themselves married. If you didn't deal with the baggage you brought from your past before you got married, now is the time to do so.

Henry Beecher expresses the beauty of recognizing the love of our parents in a new way when we become parents ourselves:

"We never know the love of the parent till we become parents ourselves. When we first bend over the cradle of our own child, God throws back the temple door, and reveals to us the sacredness and mystery of the father's and mother's love to ourselves."[1] Unfortunately, the same is true about the negative parenting of our childhood. The hurts, neglects, disappointments, or confusing messages will tend to revisit us with a vengeance as we face those situations with our own children.

Most expectant couples will benefit from some form of counseling. If the two of you come from basically intact, healthy homes, you may need only a few sessions. If either of you have a background of dysfunction, you may want to invest in a longer process and some additional individual sessions.

Counseling may not be a comfortable option for you, yet there may be parenting issues from your past that you know it would be helpful to understand before you become a parent yourself. Self-help resources are readily available. Two that I would recommend are *Living With the Love of Your Life and Loving It*[2] by Neil Clark Warren and *Getting the Love You Want*[3] by Harville Hendrix. Reading these works and writing down your reactions to them can be extremely helpful to growth, both individually and as a couple.

Get Yourself Physically Fit

Fathers, although getting and staying physically fit is essential for the mother-to-be, it is also important for you. More will be required of you in the days ahead, so take care of yourself. Do all you can to maximize your available energy.

Mothers, your body has a new purpose. It is sacred. Your body is the lifeline for your developing baby. Tracie Hotchner expresses the importance of caring for your body in her book *Pregnancy and Childbirth:*

Have you ever heard the expression "Your body is a temple"? Well, I'm not sure it was intended to be about pregnancy, but it actually does apply. Everything you eat, everything you drink, everything you breathe, everything you touch affects your growing baby. It's a big responsibility, but you may want to consider it the first of many "sacrifices" and adjustments you will have to make as a parent.[4]

Get Rest and Sleep

If you have not established healthy patterns of sleep and rest, now is the time to start. I started taking a daily nap after our first child was born and continue that habit today. I consider my nap a gift to myself, my children, my husband, and those around me. Take time to get off your feet and relax, get a nap, and provide the best conditions for nighttime sleep, even though your usual pattern may be interrupted by all that is happening in your body.

You may have difficulty sleeping at night for the first time in your life. If you are awake at night, spend the time resting and not focusing on whether you are asleep or awake. Accepting nocturnal wakefulness as an unavoidable consequence of pregnancy and not fretting about it will help you to remain at peace. I used those times for prayer.

Most books on pregnancy have a chapter on promoting good nighttime sleep. You may want to refer to such a resource for more detail. A body pillow to support the weight of your abdomen as your baby and uterus grow may be helpful. As your abdomen grows, sleeping on your back will put too much pressure on certain blood vessels and can constrict circulation for you and for the baby. The only acceptable way to sleep on your back during this time is in a reclining chair.

When sleeping in bed, you may sleep on your right side occasionally, but your *left side is recommended* to promote better blood flow to your heart and to the baby.

Eat to Nurture Your Body and Your Baby

Many of the eating habits recommended for pregnant women would be healthy for all of us all of the time. Most women accept the responsibility for their nutrition during pregnancy because of the critical nature of the possible consequences of not doing so. *Newsweek* of September 27, 1999, reviewed the scientific evidence indicating that many adult health conditions are shaped by life in the womb and are not simply due to our genetic makeup.[5]

The seriousness of nutrition during pregnancy has been emphasized for as long as I can remember. When I got pregnant, I went back to my *Obstetrics for Nurses* text. Even in that 1962 resource the recommendations were similar to those of today: four to six servings of protein per day, one quart of milk, six servings of fruits and vegetables (preferably dark green leafy and deep yellow vegetables), three to five servings of whole grains, potatoes or legumes, and adequate unsaturated fats.[6]

Hotchner lists "Food Rules" to live by for the next nine months or, even better, for the rest of your life:

- *Food is serious stuff while you're pregnant.*
- *Do not skip meals.*
- *Do not try to diet now.*
- *Pay attention to the ingredients of whatever you eat and drink.*
- *Make an extra effort to eat those foods your growing baby needs.*[7]

Whole grains and fiber are important during pregnancy. Many times whole grains and high-fiber vegetables are confused with other carbohydrates. Pregnant women may fill up on bread and pastas; however, there are very few breads or pastas that contain whole grain. Most are made from processed enriched flour, which elevates insulin levels, disrupts metabolism, and adds pounds—not adequate nutrients for baby or mother.

Whole grains contain both the inner kernel and the outer husk, which provide fiber. Examples are brown rice, whole-grain wheat, oats, rye, barley, corn, soy, millet, triticale, and breads and pastas that are labeled as whole grain. Legumes include dried peas and beans. It will be easier for you to ensure you are eating four to six servings of protein, five of vegetables, and four of high-calcium foods if you don't overload on the carbohydrates.

High vitamin C foods are also essential. However, orange juice may set off blood sugar swings and contribute to cravings.

Getting enough green leafy, yellow, and other vegetables will likely be the most difficult problem you will face in your pregnancy diet. If you eat out, this will become an even bigger challenge. Ideally you might have a large salad at lunch, an apple between meals, and two to three steamed vegetables at dinner.

A prenatal vitamin-mineral supplement is necessary. Even though a balanced diet is the best source of vitamins and minerals, in actuality there is no way to assure adequate intake for a successful pregnancy without taking a prenatal vitamin. Check with your physician to determine the best one for you.

The two basic purposes of eating for pregnancy are to nourish and to protect—to nourish yourself and your baby and to protect the baby from any harm. I have devised a silly way to remember what to focus on when choosing food for nourishment:

Pursue Pure Foods and Protein
Consume Calcium
Wallow in Water
Fine Tune Fats, Fruits, and Fiber
Vigilantly Take in Vegetables and Vitamins

To protect your baby, avoid all food or drink that could harm the baby's growth or development. Everything that goes into you will pass through your blood stream into the cells and tissue that are forming the vital organs and functions of your unborn baby.

You should avoid the following foods:[8] undercooked meats, cured meats (because of nitrites; includes cold cuts, hot dogs, ham, bacon), undercooked fish, unpasteurized milk or juices, runny eggs, soft and blue-veined cheeses, alfalfa sprouts, olestra, leftovers left too long at room temperature.

Other substances to avoid for the safety of the development of your unborn child are alcohol, nicotine, caffeine, additives, chemical sugar substitutes, and *all* drugs, whether prescription, over-the-counter, or street.

During pregnancy, alcohol should be avoided. Because there is no blood-alcohol barrier, your unborn baby will drink every drop of alcohol you do. To illustrate, how comfortable would you feel feeding your newborn a bottle of beer or a half glass of wine? Your developing baby is much smaller than a newborn, and therefore more affected by alcohol intake.

If you've inadvertently consumed one or more of these toxins at a low level, realize that consumption merely increases the risk, it does not guarantee a problem.[9]

What About Weight Gain?

Many women and men think of the pregnant woman as "getting fat" when her abdomen grows as her uterus expands and the baby develops. Women who have a history of restricting food intake to stay thin may overeat during pregnancy because they are free of society's pressure to be thin. On the other hand, women who have difficulty accepting the beauty and importance of their expanding maternal body may restrict intake of nourishment necessary during pregnancy.

At the time we had our children, we were taught that the less weight the mother-to-be gained, the better. Now we know that there can be negative consequences from low weight gain as well as from excessive weight gain. The healthy range is between twenty-five and thirty-five pounds.

You will be most successful in staying in the best weight gain range if you make sure you get the required number of servings of each of the food groups each day. Eat frequently—six small meals per day is ideal. Be accountable to someone for your eating plan and deviations from it. If you were eating adequately and not underweight before pregnancy, you need add only three to five hundred extra calories per day, and that only during the second and third trimesters. This is equivalent to two or three glasses of whole milk.

The question often asked is, "Will eating empty calories do any harm?" A good way to think about your intake of empty calories—sweets and many cereals, crackers, breads, and pastas—is that they either substitute for nutrients important for the nurturing of your baby and energy for yourself or they add extra weight to your body. The studies indicate a higher incidence of Caesarean section with excessive weight gain (more than thirty-five pounds). The uterus is a muscle. When fatty tissue collects around your uterus, uterine contractions may be less effective during labor and delivery. Obviously, the occasional indulgence is not likely to have noticeable consequences. Still, some caution is necessary. If you are one of those women who can take in all the servings of the needed food groups and still eat the empty carbos, enjoy! However, if you are like most of us, the discipline of a prescribed eating plan will be well worth the effort.

All women come to pregnancy with a history of eating patterns and habits. Pregnancy is a wonderful time to confirm healthy eating habits and to discard unhealthy ways of thinking about your body and food.

Exercise to Prepare Your Body for Labor and Delivery
Commitment to exercise needs to be accompanied by manageable goals and a lot of grace in order to be successful long-term. My commitment to daily exercise started during my first pregnancy. My children laugh at my exercise routine, but it has worked for me. It starts with a fifteen-minute morning workout with a rope pulley that I purchased for 99 cents thirty-two years ago. A number of years later, I added an aerobic workout that I do on a trampoline-type exerciser, or my husband and I walk in the evening for twenty-five minutes. Even though my goal is to exercise every day, there are many days I do not. If I fulfill my goal four to five times per week, I am successful. There have been weeks when workouts have not been possible, but then I start back as soon as I can.

You may be well established in an exercise routine that works for you. If so, only adaptation may be necessary. Your body's needs during pregnancy are different than they are at any other time. Any jarring exercise like jogging, skiing, horseback riding, or a contact sport is best replaced by brisk walking, swimming, or other aerobic activity approved by your physician. At high altitudes, exercise with caution. Sit-ups or exercises that pull the abdominal muscles are not recommended during pregnancy. More important than aerobic exercises are the relaxation techniques and exercises that prepare you for labor and delivery.

Think of the task of preparing your body to perform its valuable function of producing a new life as similar to the training before an upcoming competition of an athlete who hopes to win at her sport. Labor and delivery will be physically demanding. Prepare your body; you will be grateful that you did.

Aerobic excercise can best be guided by your physician or the director of your pregnancy exercise program. *Relaxation exercise* helps you learn to have control of the action of relaxation even if you cannot control the feelings that interfere with relaxation. Together and separately, you can learn to put yourselves and each other into a state of deep relaxation. Husbands can help their wives relax during labor. For guidance, buy an audio relaxation tape or refer to the steps in *Your Pregnancy Companion* by Janis Graham, pages 176–77.

Exercises for labor and delivery are pictured and described in more detail in Dr. William and Martha Sears' *The Pregnancy Book,* pages 169–80 and in most pregnancy resources. The *Kegal, PC,* or *Pubococcygeus muscle exercises,* which strengthen your pelvic floor muscles, are the most important for labor and delivery. Tighten and relax those muscles one to two hundred times per day. You can do these anytime and anywhere, and no one will know. To determine that you are tightening the correct muscle, sit on the toilet, spread your legs, and stop and start urination several times. *Squatting and tailor sitting* are not only valuable preparation, but are also helpful during labor. *Pelvic tilt exercises* relieve back pressure and help prepare your body and the position of the baby for birth. You align or straighten your back and then relax it without sagging. These can be done lying on your back with your knees bent during the first four months and standing, sitting, or on all fours throughout your pregnancy. Three types of *breathing*—slow, regular, relaxed breathing for between contractions, deep abdominal breathing during contractions and a series of short pants punctuated by blows outward for intense contractions and slowing down the urge to push—would be best practiced daily.

Care for Each Other and Your Relationship

Build Your Relationship

As the expectant *father,* be diligent about staying connected. Being emotionally available and empathizing with your wife's fluctuating feelings without taking her reactions personally or getting defensive will make a *huge* difference in your marriage. Physically relieving her of or assisting her with projects around the house will help her be able to take care of her body and your developing baby. In addition to bonding with and being intimately involved in the care of your newborn child, *the greatest contribution you can make is caring for your child's mother.* Start with a simple formula: every day take fifteen minutes to

- connect with her and with what she is feeling,
- compliment her and express your appreciation,
- share your concerns and thoughts,
- kiss her warmly without leading to sex, and ask her how she needs you to help.

As the expectant *mother,* take time to show your interest in your husband's life. What are his pressures, concerns, and thoughts in general and in relation to your pregnancy and upcoming parenting roles and tasks? Learn now to take responsibility for letting him know what you need from him rather than nagging or complaining about his lack of helpfulness, which will only make him feel bad about himself or angry with you and create distance.

Together plan time for the two of you and keep that commitment to couple time after the baby is born, even if it is limited to just fifteen minutes a day. My husband's and my book *Men and Sex*[10] teaches the principles of intimacy in marriage that go far beyond sex and are applicable for practice in building your relationship during and after pregnancy.

Keep Your Sex Life Alive

Even though sex is the way to pregnancy, pregnancy can be the demise of a couple's sex life. Fatigue, hormonal changes, nausea, physical discomforts, difficulty accepting the woman's bodily changes, unbased fears of harming the baby, or other emotional or physical issues may get in the way. On the other hand, pregnancy may heighten sexual enjoyment and activity because there is no need for contraception, and the bonding of the pregnancy brings a new desire for intimacy.

To keep your sexual life alive during and after pregnancy, plan quality times. You will increase the enjoyment of sex without fatigue, and will increase the frequency of intimate moments. Plan a lighthearted time to practice getting your bodies into various positions without actually having intercourse, just to see what will work in the later months of pregnancy. Keep sex mutually satisfying. It will never be great if one is demanding sex and the other is submitting out of duty. Sex isn't about meeting needs; it's about sharing fullness, intimacy, love, and care. Sex isn't the machine of marriage, it is the lubricant. Without the lubricant, the machine won't work for long.

Build Your Spiritual Connection

As part of your fifteen-minute connecting time each day, read a Bible verse or a short devotional, or say a short prayer together. Study Bibles and programs for couples are readily available. If these require more time commitment than you are likely to be able to manage successfully, start more simply with a flip calendar that has an inspirational thought or Scripture verse for each day. Use the prayer suggestions in the monthly chapters that follow in this book. Take time to know God.

Many couples long for something more than the busyness of the life they are living. The husband may have tried to settle his uneasiness by pursuing more frequent sex with his wife or increasing his performance and productivity at work. The wife may complain that he isn't the spiritual leader of their home. She may become more involved in Christian activities in an attempt to fill her hunger for spiritual intimacy. Whether you are the husband or the wife who has felt this nudge for something more, listen and respond to your craving without placing demands on your spouse to meet that need. Invite your spouse to share spiritual communion with you as you take responsibility for planning for those times.

Pregnancy is a profound time of life. Most of us are pregnant for a very small percentage of our lifetime. Cherish this time. When I had to have a hysterectomy, the two losses I had to face were that I would never be pregnant again and I would never again breastfeed. Neither were realistic possibilities for me anymore, but both had been deeply meaningful, short-lived life experiences that I had celebrated.

As you approach the end of your pregnancy, you may wish you could shorten the time it takes to grow a baby, but remember that it takes most of us that long to really be ready. Don't rush delivery. Savor this time to the end.

> She is clothed with strength and dignity, and she laughs with no fear of the future. When she speaks, her words are wise, and kindness is the rule when she gives instruction. She carefully watches all that goes on in her household and does not have to bear the consequences of laziness. Her children stand and bless her. Her husband praises her: "There are many virtuous and capable women in the world, but you surpass them all!"
>
> PROVERBS 31:25-29, NLT

Lord, through all generations you have been our
home!
Before the mountains were created, before you made
the earth and the world, you are God, without
beginning or end.
Teach us to make the most of our time, so that we can
grow in wisdom.
Let us see your miracles again; let our children see
your glory at work. And may the Lord our God
show us his approval and make our efforts successful. Yes, make our efforts successful!

PSALM 90: 1-2, 12, 16-17, NLT

On Parenting

Quality is never an accident; it is always the result of high
intention, sincere effort, intelligent direction and skillful
execution; it represents the wise choice of many alternatives"
(Willa A. Foster).[1]

We must be proactive about parenting if we are going to raise
children to be persons of integrity, internal strength, wise discernment, and trust in God.

We will raise well-adjusted, responsible children only when
we parent with clear expectations, high standards, and unconditional warmth, and we teach children discernment as we
empower them to make good choices. If, as we raise our chil-

dren, we teach them to blindly obey, we raise people without an inner sense of right and wrong and no awareness of how to listen to their conscience. They are open to follow either good or bad authorities if they follow authority with blind obedience. Yet, if we raise our children with no boundaries and no values or morals, they will listen only to their inner selves and do whatever "feels good" or whatever seems "right in their own eyes."

My husband and I have taught parenting classes in various settings since our oldest children were young. Teaching others and parenting so that negative patterns are not passed from one generation to the next is an awesome but rewarding responsibility.

For Our Children

Father, hear us, we are praying,
Hear the words our hearts are saying,
We are praying for our children.

Keep them from the powers of evil,
From the secret, hidden peril,
From the whirlpool that would suck them,
From the treacherous quicksand, pluck them.
From the wordling's hollow gladness
From the sting of faithless sadness
Holy Father, save our children.

Through life's troubled waters steer them,
Through life's bitter battle cheer them,
Father, Father, be Thou near them.

Read the language of our longing,
Read the wordless pleadings thronging,
Holy Father, for our children.

And wherever they may bide,
Lead them home at eventide.

Amy Carmichael[2]

Without God, we cannot change our parenting. Being a parent is the most awesome of all responsibilities. You can't do it alone. Gather people around you. Allow others to mentor you and be mirrors to you of what they see. We need the perspective of God's family as well as the strength of God in us. "'Not by might nor by power, but by My Spirit,' says the Lord of hosts" (Zechariah 4:6, NASB).

Adjustments of Parenting

The first adjustment of parenting is *suspension of your needs and desires*. Parenting requires the best of Christlike character. When we become parents, we suspend momentary gratification of our own needs and rights for those of our children, even as Christ did for us.

> If you've gotten anything at all out of following Christ, if his love has made any difference in your life, if being in a community of the Spirit means anything to you ... don't push your way to the front.... Put yourself aside.... Think of yourselves the way Christ Jesus thought of himself. He had equal status with God but didn't think so much of himself that he had to cling to the advantages of that status. Not at all. When the time came, he set aside the privileges of deity and took on the status of a slave, became human!... He didn't claim special privileges. Instead, he lived a selfless, obedient life.
>
> PHILIPPIANS 2:1-7, THE MESSAGE

The sacrifices of parenting have already started with your pregnancy. Your lives have changed. The mother's body has made significant adjustments and sacrifices for the benefit of your unborn child. Parenting will continue that process of change.

Giving of yourselves for your children doesn't mean you don't take care of yourselves. You must. Christ gave generously, yet even He went away from the crowd to rest and to pray after He had given of Himself. When your infant needs to eat you won't be able to say, "Not now, honey. I'm too tired." But after you have fed him or her, take time to rest.

The second adjustment of parenting is *the relentless responsibility*. You can't leave your job at night; you are on duty twenty-four hours a day, seven days a week. You can never relinquish your responsibility. Even when someone else cares for your child, you will have the ultimate responsibility for that care.

Other adjustments will be inevitable. You will learn to anticipate and be more deliberate about life. You will no longer be able to say, "Let's go to a movie tonight." You will have to plan.

Adult conversation will become a rarity. Once children start moving around and talking, adult conversation occurs only after their bedtime. We experienced that this summer on our family vacation with two toddler grandchildren. We had so much fun, yet it was very different than in past years when we were seven adults.

These adjustments will be much easier if you have had previous exposure to babies and young children. Offer to work in the nursery at church. Baby-sit for friends. This will ease your transition into parenthood.

Although parenting requires change, the gains far outweigh the losses. Parenting will make you a better person. I am convinced that as we bond with our babies, love our children who are flesh of our flesh, listen to them, and adapt our ways to what is best for their growth and development, we become better people. In many ways we truly become adult in the sense described in M. Scott Peck's book *The Road Less Traveled*.[3] We learn to delay immediate gratification, sometimes referred to as short-term pain, for long-term gain. And even though we may not see the rewards of our parenting for a long, long time, children bring daily joy and fulfillment.

Styles of Parenting

When my husband and I started teaching parenting in the early seventies, we developed three parenting models to help describe the various theories. The titles given to these models in many parenting books are Authoritarian (we call it Strongly Parent-Directed), Permissive, and Authoritative (Come-Alongside).

Understanding the styles and expected outcomes of each approach will be helpful to you in making decisions about handling your child.

Strongly Parent-Directed parenting is firm and punitive. Authoritarian parents set up demands and commands and make their children's decisions for them. The style is prescriptive or rule-oriented with an emphasis on obedience to absolute standards. Many times parents will take an adversarial role in relation to their children; the children often feel their parents are not on their side. The children are expected to conform to their parents rather than having the parent adapt to the uniqueness of each child. The parents are dominant, and children are kept in their place. The prescriptiveness of this model is very inviting to new parents, and compliant, easy-to-manage children are an immediate gratification. The ultimate outcome of this style of parenting is of significant concern, however.

Children of authoritarian parents can become compliant and

dependent, withdrawn, distrustful, discontent and irritable, limited in their sense of responsibility and achievement, socially undeveloped, and lacking in spontaneity, curiosity, affection, and originality.

Permissive parenting is chosen by parents who see their relationship to their children as determined by the children, rather than seeing themselves as role models or agents responsible for shaping their children's behavior. Permissive parents are highly tolerant of all child behavior and consider establishment of schedules, assertion of parental authority, and expectations of maturity as detrimental to their children's psychological well-being. They offer their children little or no guidance for growth and development. Such parents are at the opposite end of the spectrum from controlling parents. They provide few controls, and boundaries and expectations are unclear. Their children are expected to make their own decisions and often are allowed to run the home. Permissive parents are often insecure and may be intimidated by their children, while the lack of boundaries and parental involvement in such a parenting style leaves children feeling unsafe and insecure.

Children of permissive parents can become dependent, immature and self-centered, lacking in self-control, limited in feelings of social responsibility, impulsive, aggressive and angry, and low achievers.

Come-Alongside parenting facilitates children's independence through appropriate assistance, encouragement, and limit setting. The parents who practice this style are loving, firm, and understanding, with high, clear, and age-appropriate expectations. Structure and boundaries, which are based on the natural rhythm of each child, are clear and consistent but allow plenty of room for the expression and choices of each child. Another way of describing the parenting practices of this model is that the children have no doubt who is in charge, but they don't feel hemmed in with arbitrary restrictions. Children feel empowered to make choices and learn decision-making skills. Parents are the trainers, teachers, and coaches. The parents and the children are on the same team. Parents are involved advocates for their children who value disciplined conformity, yet are willing to defer their needs for the best interests of their children. Such parents guide their children to fit society's expectations, while respecting the individual personality of each child. Self-control and self-discipline are prominent characteristics of these parents.

Come-alongside parents practice mutual respect and promote decision making, critical thinking, and independence. The parents are there, carefully observant, as they allow their children to move out on their own. The children gradually progress, from complete dependence upon the parents at birth to sufficient independence by the time they are ready to leave home.

Come-alongside parents must be careful to balance the messages they send to their children, so that they are best suited for the development of the children. In a sense, there are two competing messages: initially the newborn needs to know "Your needs will always be taken care of," and "I will always be here for you." As children mature, parents begin to introduce the reality that "You won't always get everything you want," and "You can comfort (or do it) yourself." The children must gain the security that their parents will always be there for them at the same time that these children are gradually learning to be self-reliant. Come-alongside parents can be represented as crouching behind their children, with hands on either side, but not touching them, ready to support them if they lose their balance as they learn to walk.

Come-alongside parents have the happiest children. Children of come-alongside parents often are self-reliant, self-controlled, explorative, content, assertive, socially responsible, and academically successful.

Out of necessity we must bring up one more parenting style—one that isn't an option. **Negligent or Abusive parenting** isn't likely to be practiced by anyone caring enough to read this book. Negligent and abusive parents abdicate their parental responsibilities. What *they* want or feel or do is more important than the impact of their feelings, reactions, desires, and actions on their children. We are *never* to sacrifice the physical, emotional, or spiritual needs of the child for the parent.

Let's look at examples of these parenting approaches applied:

Example 1: A mother walks in on her toddler climbing a precarious chair to reach a toy that has been put on a shelf. The strongly directive mother reprimands the child for an unsafe action, takes the child off of the chair, and does not let the child get the toy. The permissive mother gets the toy for the child. The come-alongside mother holds the chair for the child, helping the child to get the toy for himself and teaching him how to safely get the toy. The negligent mother isn't even aware of what the child is doing, so the child falls and hurts himself. The abusive mother reacts in rage and pulls the child by the arm or slaps the child.

Example 2: A two-year-old starts resisting his parents' choice of clothing. The strongly directive parent tells the child that these are the clothes he will be wearing and punishes him until he puts them on. The permissive parent lets the child wear whatever she wants to go out in the yard to play, even if it is her special new outfit. Alternatively, the permissive parent tries to talk the child into wearing the chosen outfit, but gives in one time and uses force another. The come-alongside parent selects several acceptable outfits and lets the child choose one, teaching about what type of clothing is suitable for different situations and reinforcing the child's move into independence. The negligent parent isn't even involved. The child may or may not get dressed. The abusive parent verbally or physically hurts the child to force him to wear the clothes selected.

Ephesians 6 teaches the importance of children obeying and honoring their parents, and emphasizes how we as parents are to elicit our children's obedience and honor:

> Don't make your children angry by the way you treat them. Rather, bring them up with the discipline and instruction approved by the Lord.
>
> EPHESIANS 6:4, NLT

Positive parenting includes believing in your children, being their advocate, validating them, delighting in them, anticipating their needs, empathizing with them, training them, and being consistent with them.[4] The products of positive parenting are children characterized by uniqueness, competence, significance, virtue, and power. Positive results of parenting may be possible only when you are willing to change yourself, not your children. When you change who you are, your manner with your children will change, and your children will acquire the qualities that you wish to instill in them.

Parenting is a ministry, far more than a mere job. Parenting will never be easy. Pray for God to bless you with a passion for parenting. There will be times when your only prayer may be similar to that of Sam Meier: "I pray every morning. My prayers consist of one word: HELP. That's it—over and out. And then I get up and do something." (Sam Meier)[5]

Or you may pray this prayer that came to us via e-mail:

I want to thank you, Lord, for being
Close to me so far this day.
With your help, I haven't been impatient,
Lost my temper, been grumpy,
Judgmental, or envious of anyone.
But I will be getting out of bed in a minute,
And I think I will really need your help then. Amen.

Or, more seriously, you might pray with Thomas Aquinas:

Give me, O Lord, a steadfast heart, which no unworthy affection may drag downwards; give me an unconquered heart, which no unworthy purpose may tempt aside. Bestow on me also, O Lord my God, understanding to know you, diligence to seek you, wisdom to find you, and a faithfulness that may finally embrace you, through Jesus Christ our Lord. Amen.[6]

Spiritual Formation of Your Child

Parents are instructed throughout Scripture to model and to develop their children's relationship with God. John the Baptist is said to have received the Holy Spirit while in his mother's womb. You don't have to wait to plan and pray for the spiritual development of your child; you can start that focus right now.

Pray that all your children will be taught of the Lord; and the well-being of your children will be great.

ADAPTED FROM ISAIAH 54:13, NASB

Dedicate Your Child to God

When you bring your infant to God through the formality of baptism or dedication, you are committing yourself to bringing your child to Christ and teaching him the Christian faith and life.

For I know the one in whom I trust, and I am sure that he is able to guard what I have entrusted to him until the day of his return. Hold on to the pattern of right teaching you learned from me. And remember to live in the faith and love that you have in Christ Jesus. With the help of the Holy Spirit who lives within us, carefully guard what has been entrusted to you.

2 TIMOTHY 1:12-14, NLT

Choose a Place of Worship

Becoming part of a church provides you with a caring community, a sense of tradition, structure to practice your faith, and an opportunity to worship God. The community you choose for worship will also share the values that you hope to impart to your children; you won't have to do your job alone.

Come, let us worship and bow down. Let us kneel before the Lord our maker, for he is our God. We are the people he watches over, the sheep under his care.

PSALM 95:6-7, NLT

Model Christ's Love to Your Children and to Others

Children form their view of God from their parents. As your children are able to trust you, they will be able to form a trusting relationship with God. As you live what you believe and teach, your children will embrace your spiritual instructions. You will have a powerful influence on your children's relationship with God.

> Fix your thoughts on what is true and honorable and right. Think about things that are excellent and worthy of praise. Keep putting into practice all you learned from me and heard from me and saw me doing, and the God of peace will be with you.
>
> PHILIPPIANS 4:8-9, NLT

> Give to your children; don't expect them to give to you. Little children don't pay for their parents' food. It's the other way around; parents supply food for their children. I will gladly spend myself and all I have for your spiritual good.
>
> 2 CORINTHIANS 12:14-15, NLT

Share Biblical Songs and Stories With Your Child

Children are receptive to learning about God and comforted by the sense of His care from a very young age. You can have a powerful impact on their spiritual development by sharing the biblical teachings early in their lives.

You can start reading the *Baby Bible Storybook*[7] by Robin Currie right at birth. The *Bible Storybook*[8] by Georgie Adams has longer stories to read as children get older. Our children started to read the first book to our two-year-old grandson at birth. Now he says the prayer at the end of each story by memory and loves the familiarity of the baby book, but is more intrigued by the longer stories of Georgie Adams' book.

And you must love the Lord your God with all your heart, all your soul, and all your strength. And you must commit yourselves wholeheartedly to these commands I am giving you today. Repeat them again and again to your children.

DEUTERONOMY 6:5-7, NLT

Teach Your Child to Pray

Pray with your child. Communication within the family is important to building family relationships; likewise, talking with God as a family will build the family's relationship with God. Teach little prayer rituals like grace at mealtime and bedtime prayers, as well as spontaneous prayers. Take a moment to thank God or encourage your child to thank God for something special in your day. Ask God for help at difficult moments.

When our children were school-age, we placed an erasable prayer board right by our kitchen table, the common location for sharing prayer concerns. On one side of the board we dated and listed prayer requests. On the other side of the board we noted when and how the request was answered.

A Small Child's Book of Prayers[9] includes many of the old traditional prayers, revised appropriately. For example, the "if I should die" phrase in the prayer I learned to pray at bedtime has been replaced with a positive, less fear-inducing phrase.

Praying with and for your children can be a means of open communication between you and them. As they reach the difficult teen years, you might write down your prayers for them as a way of letting them know you care about and understand their situations of life.

A Prayer

Help me to the stature of good parenthood:

I pray that I may let my child live his own life and not the one I wish I had lived. Guard me against burdening him with doing what I failed to do.

Help me see today's missteps in perspective against the long road he must go, and give me patience with his pace, lest I—in my impatience—force him into rebellion, retreat or anxiety.

Give me the precious wisdom of knowing when to smile at the small mischiefs of his age and when to give him the haven of firmness against the impulses which in his heart he fears and cannot master.

In time of needed punishment give me a warm heart and a gentle voice so that he may feel the rule of order is his friend and clasp it to himself. Help me to let him know in advance what the consequences of his actions will be.

Help me to hear the anguish of his heart through the din of angry words or across the gulf of brooding silence and having heard, give me the grace to bridge the gap between us with understanding warmth before speaking my own quick retorts. Stay my tongue from all that would chill his confiding in me.

I pray that I may raise my voice more in joy at what he is than in vexation for what he is not, so that each day he may grow in sureness of himself. Help me to hold him with such warmth as will give him friendliness toward fellow man; strongly on his way.

Dr. Marion Durfee[10]

We're pregnant! Joy unspeakable! Lord, we give You thanks and praise for allowing us the awesome responsibility to be called "mother" and "father." Prepare us for parenthood both physically and emotionally. Help me, as a mother-to-be, through nausea, sleepiness, and craving for crazy foods. Bless and protect the little one in my womb. Help me, as husband, to understand the adjustments my wife is having to make because of her pregnancy. Lord, we're trusting you for a safe delivery. Amen.[1]

The First Month: Sharing the News

Excitement, anticipation, and adjustment are typical feelings during the first month of pregnancy. You may have "known" almost immediately that you were pregnant, or much of this first month may have passed before you suspected and confirmed your suspicions. Either way, it's big news!

The drama of conception and the growth of each new human being from just two tiny cells—an egg from the female, called an ovum, and a sperm from the male—is a wonderful demonstration of God's creative and scientific power. At the same time, your body's response to this miniscule new life has challenged the reasoning of the best scientists and has wreaked havoc on many a pregnant woman's body. How can a process so small be so powerful? The wonderment of that question will continue throughout your child's life.

The Growing Baby

At this stage your developing baby is called an embryo, "a gentle euphemism related to the Greek verb form 'to be full of life.'"[2] Indeed, this is the month when this new life is forming and building its basic parts.

When the sperm from the male and ovum from the female—each an incomplete cell—unite, they form a cell that is complete and can begin to grow. This newly formed cell contains all the material from which the baby gets its inheritance: whether it is a boy or girl, what he or she will look like, and the basis for his or her capabilities and personality characteristics. This cell divides into two cells, the two into four, and so on, with the cells initially dividing at a very rapid pace.

It takes three to five days for this cluster of cells to find its way to the thick, soft lining of the uterus. As the new life settles into the lining of the uterus, it finds a bed and food for itself. The tiny cluster of cells, smaller than a grain of rice, is the beginning of your little baby, with all its makings intricately designed by God.

Perhaps now would be a good time to pray a prayer of praise for the miracle of conception. Put this in your own words, or use these words I have written for you:

Dear Heavenly Father,
    You are the giver of life. You have blessed us beyond our

dreams. Thank You for the gift of conception. It is amazing to imagine all parts of our baby are already present in that rice-sized person. We praise You for the miracle of conception and thank You specifically for our baby. Amen.

By the end of the first month, all the internal organs, the backbone, and the spinal cord are forming. The heart actually begins to beat, even though it won't be heard for many more weeks. No eyes, nose, or external ears are visible. Small buds that will eventually become arms and legs are present. The baby's body begins to take on a distinct C shape with a visible front and back and left and right. This is the beginning of a critical period of formation because the baby's organs and systems are developing so rapidly.

Pray a prayer for the design and formation of your baby:

Dear Father, Our Creator,

You know exactly how our baby's cells are multiplying. You are not only the giver of life; You are also the designer. We commit every intricate detail of our baby's body to You. Strengthen that tiny, tiny heart, which has started to beat. Mold every organ. We thank You for Your tender care. In Jesus' name, Amen.

Changes in the Mother-to-Be

Your uterus, your baby's home for the next nine months, is an amazingly vital body part. It changes in pregnancy from an almost solid organ about the size of your closed fist into a large, thin-walled sac that maintains a constant temperature and grows as the baby grows without disturbing the function of other vital organs. It weighs about one ounce before pregnancy and slightly more than two pounds by the end of the pregnancy.

The uterus does much more than house your baby for these months. Cells that come from the fertilized egg attach to the wall of the uterus and grow to form the placenta, or what is often referred to as the afterbirth. Cells from the placenta tap into the mother's blood supply to bring nourishment to the baby and carry away waste. Everything the mother takes into her body, even something so small as an aspirin, will travel through to the baby and can potentially affect its development.

The amniotic fluid, or "bag of waters," is produced in the uterus. It surrounds the baby so that the walls of the uterus don't cramp it, allows the baby to move around, maintains a constant temperature, provides fluid for the baby, and cushions the baby against injury—it is an excellent shock absorber. This liquid is not stagnant. It is constantly being replaced.

Picture God putting His arms of protection around you and your baby as you say this prayer:

Dear God,

Even as you have designed the uterus to carry and protect our growing baby, we are confident of Your protection and care for us. We picture the placenta forming to nurture our baby and the amniotic fluid surrounding and cushioning him. In the same way we think of Your Spirit surrounding us and our baby and cushioning us all from the bumps of life. We praise You for Your presence in our lives. Amen.

You may also have noticed the changes taking place in your vagina and breasts. The vagina becomes more elastic and increases in blood supply, causing a bluish or dark violet coloring of the genitals. This color change is often an early sign of pregnancy. The breasts become fuller and more sensitive, and the nipples darken.

All the changes taking place in your body will naturally affect your feelings. When the baby's development is at a critical period of rapid growth, you are likely to experience fatigue. Fatigue is a sign that your body needs more rest. If you can get that nap, you will replenish the energy supplies that are being drained by the baby. To reduce fatigue, make certain you are taking your prenatal vitamin as often as instructed, avoiding simple carbohydrates, and taking in enough of each of your essential food groups.

Take time alone to rest and pray. Jesus taught His followers to handle the busy-ness of life and to get a perspective on priorities through spending time alone with Him.

And He said to them, "Come away by yourselves to a lonely place and rest a while."

MARK 6:31, NASB

Morning sickness, a misnomer for nausea during pregnancy, may trouble you at any or all times of the day. It can zap your joy and turn early pregnancy into day-to-day survival. If nausea is severe, medical intervention may be necessary. The complex hormonal changes, the physiological stress a pregnant woman's body endures, and the stress of the many emotions associated with pregnancy are all thought to influence morning sickness. But take heart: nausea and vomiting are actually believed to be signs of a healthy pregnancy, because they are associated with high levels of human chorionic gonadotropin (hCG), a hormone produced by the placenta that keeps the pregnancy on course. Why some women feel the effects of this hormone—levels of which are highest between the eighth and twelfth weeks—while others do not, is unknown.

As a graduate student at UCLA, I researched nausea in pregnancy. I discovered an interesting correlation between crying and nausea. Women who estimated they cried 170 to 365 times per year reported almost no nausea during pregnancy; women who cried infrequently varied in their reports of nausea. You may wonder why crying might reduce nausea.

Although lack of crying does not cause nausea, crying releases stress in the body. It is a let-down response. Nausea is a stress response. When you cry, you help your body shift its nervous system control and let go of the stress reaction.

If you are a person who tends to keep stress bottled inside you, you might rent a video that will trigger your tears. I used to watch "Little House on the Prairie" with Kristine, our youngest daughter, when she was little. Inevitably, I would cry. Our oldest daughter remembers those times and just recently gave me the video series of "Little House on the Prairie." If I ever have the need to cry, I have my resources ready.

Your need to cry may be based on deeper issues. Seeing a counselor for a few sessions may be a valuable outlet for any internal conflict. Many parishes and churches have lay counseling programs if therapy is not a financial possibility for you. Take time to listen to your body and your feelings. Whatever helps you let your tears flow to release emotions and stress, try it.

There are ways other than crying to encourage your nervous system to let down and to help reduce nausea. Sleep and salivation are two things that are particularly beneficial in reducing the nausea of pregnancy. You will probably find that you are less nauseated when you are more rested. Getting up in the morning, because your body is shifting from relaxation into action, often triggers nausea. Nibbling on a cracker or rice cake, sucking on a lemon drop or mint, or chewing gum to stimulate salivation before you get up may decrease morning sickness by activating your gastrointestinal system, with its let-down mechanism. Eating small amounts frequently throughout the day keeps salivation stimulated and also stabilizes your blood sugar, to counteract all-day nausea.

The changes you are experiencing are evidence that your body is adjusting and assuming the remarkable function of producing a new life. You can be proud. Share with your husband, family, and friends all the little and not-so-little nuances you feel.

Decision of the Month

Sharing the News

The first month you may have many thoughts about decisions that will be important to your pregnancy, childbirth, and parenting. The first decision will likely be whom do we tell first? How and when do we tell? When is it public knowledge?

Our son Greg and his wife Carrie, are the parents of our first grandchild, Kevin. To announce their pregnancy, they invited us to go out to dinner with them. They brought us each a small gift bag, and when Cliff and I reached into our bags, we pulled out T-shirts. Mine said "Grandma" and Cliff's said "Grandpa." What an overwhelming moment of surprise! I'll always remember the hesitation—Grandma?—and then exclamation—"Grandma!"

A second surprise announcement came from our daughter Julene and her husband John a little less than a year later. Because of some past medical treatments, the likelihood of them being able to have their own children was in question. At brunch with our entire family, Julene said she wanted to give a special toast to little Kevin, her nephew. She ended her toast by saying, "We've been thinking about a gift that would be just right for Kevin's first birthday. We think we have the perfect gift for him: a cousin."

You and your spouse might want to talk about how, when, and to whom you want to tell the news. The two of you likely will have differences of opinion regarding this and many other decisions. Discussing your thoughts and feelings and really listening to one another often will help you to bring your individual ideas together to create an even better plan.

Deciding When to Tell Your Other Children
If you already have children, keep in mind that your baby's siblings may or may not be happy about the news. Just think how you might feel if your husband brought a mistress home. He might reassure you that this other person would not affect his love for you and that he was sure that it would be fun for you to have another woman around. Still, you would find this upsetting! Bringing home a new baby can cause much the same feeling in your other children.

When and how to tell siblings depends on their age and your sense of their readiness for this huge change in their lives. It is usually suggested that you wait until you are through the more risky first trimester before you involve your other children. It is then important to include them in as much of the process as you deem appropriate. Give older children a role, like talking to the baby, singing to her, kissing Mommy's tummy, or helping to choose a name. Encourage each child to express his or her feelings. Adele Faber and Elaine Mazlish's book *Siblings Without Rivalry*[3] gives some great suggestions for how to handle this tricky situation.

Pray a prayer of praise for the good news, and ask for sensitivity in sharing it. Use your own words, or these words I have written for you:

> We want to shout our good news to everyone, Dear God, yet we know for some of our childless friends our pregnancy will be a painful reminder of what they are missing. Lord, give us sensitivity in timing and words. Bless them, O Giver of Life. Also give us sensitivity in including our children in this joyful transition in our lives. May we continue to validate our love for them and their special importance to us at this time when they may feel confused. Thank You for Your guidance. In Jesus' name, Amen.

Tasks, Hopes, and Dreams for the Month

Selecting Your Health Care Practitioner

An early task of pregnancy is the selection of a health professional to provide your prenatal care and manage your labor and delivery. You may have already completed this process. If not, now is the time.

The professional who provides your health care could be a family practitioner who is a medical doctor or a doctor of osteopathy; an obstetrician; a nurse practitioner or midwife; or a prenatal clinic with a variety of professionals serving you. An obstetrician is most specialized and will tend to focus on the medical aspects of your pregnancy and pending childbirth. A midwife will utilize more natural birthing techniques and will be open to alternative approaches to care. Be informed not only about the qualifications of the professional you choose but also about that person's or facility's reputation and hospital affiliation.

Call your insurance provider to obtain a list of professionals who offer prenatal and maternity care and are part of your plan. Once you have a list of possible providers, you can ask others about those available to you.

Get referrals from other couples in your community who have had a baby recently or from medical professionals. A great resource for an honest referral is a nurse or healthcare person who works in the maternity unit of the hospital you are considering for your labor and delivery. This person will know from behind the scenes who he or she would choose.

The Internet is another resource for checking out referral sources. You can write the International Childbirth Education Association at P.O. Box 20048, Minneapolis, MN 55420, or call them at 612-854-8660. Their web site can be found at www.icea.org. For a midwife referral, contact the American College of Nurse-Midwives, 818 Connecticut Avenue NW, Suite 900, Washington, D.C. 20006, or call them at 202-728-9860. Their web site can be found at www.midwife.org.

Visit the hospitals or birthing centers and call the offices of the practitioners you are considering. You will want to assess how well the hospital and practitioner fit your needs.

Is the location convenient, in case you should have to be there quickly? The hospital we used to delivery Julene and Gregory, our first two children, was twenty to twenty-five minutes away from where we were living, but the obstetrician offered his services free to us as students at Fuller Theological Graduate School of Psychology. The free service took precedence over the distance.

What is the hospital setup for labor and delivery? Will you deliver and recover in the same room you are in for labor? What electronic monitoring is used? What if you have concerns?

Consider asking the practitioner how many of your appointments will actually be with him or her, and his or her views on weight gain and nutrition during pregnancy, coached labor and delivery, pain relief methods, and criteria for and frequency of Caesarean sections.

Whomever you choose, never allow yourself to be intimidated. Listen to your intuition, and let the care provider know your feelings. Pray for wisdom, discernment, and strength to pursue the necessary information to choose a health care practitioner who is best for you. Pray that with a loving attitude, you will have the strength to stand up for what you believe is right.

Calculating Your Due Date

There are two ways to calculate the length of your pregnancy and determine your due date. The first is usually the due date given by your physician and is calculated from the first day of your last normal menstrual period. Based on this method your due date is 280 days after your last menstrual period. Using the second method of calculation, your due date is determined by the actual date of conception. By this method, the due date is 266 to 267 days from the day of conception.

For the sake of clarity, the nine months of pregnancy are arbitrarily divided into three stages, or trimesters. The first three months comprise the first trimester, the second three months the second trimester, and the last three months the third trimester.

Prayers and Scripture

O Lord Almighty, God of Israel, I have been bold enough to pray this prayer because you have revealed that you will build a house for me—an eternal dynasty! For you are God, O Sovereign Lord. Your words are truth, and you have promised these good things to me, your servant. And now, may it please you to bless me and my family so that our dynasty may continue forever before you. For when you grant a blessing to your servant, O Sovereign Lord, it is an eternal blessing!

2 SAMUEL 7:27-29, NLT

Father, we ask your blessing upon our family and our home. Put your shield of protection around all who live and visit here, guarding us from evil and from harm. May your holy presence abide here.

I speak Aaron's priestly blessing over my family: "The Lord bless you and keep you; the Lord make his face shine upon you and be gracious to you; the Lord turn his face toward you and give you peace" (Numbers 6:22). Amen.

Quin Sherrer and Ruthanne Garlock[4]

Family Prayer Journal

A new pregnancy brings with it so much change, it sometimes can be overshelming. Quiet time for prayer and meditation will help you center on God and His strength in you. Increased comfort and peace will follow. Each month use these suggestions to record your prayers, so that you can release your concerns to God and give praise when these concerns are answered.

- Focus on recognizing God's power in your life and relinquishing your will to Him.
- Express thanks and joy to God.
- Praise Him for prayers that have been answered this month.
- Offer praises and requests related to your baby's growth and development this month.
- Pray for each family member.
- Pray for the decisions and tasks of this month.
- Pray for forgiveness and guidance.

Oh yes, you shaped me first inside, then out;
   you formed me in my mother's womb.
I thank you, High God—you're breathtaking!
   Body and soul, I am marvelously made!
   I worship in adoration—what a creation!
You know me inside and out,
   you know every bone in my body;
You know exactly how I was made, bit by bit,
   how I was sculpted from nothing into something.
Like an open book, you watched me grow from
   conception to birth;
   all stages of my life were spread out before you,
The days of my life all prepared
   before I'd even lived one day.

PSALM 139:13-16, THE MESSAGE

The Second Month:
Caring for Yourself and Your Baby

The growing reality of the pregnancy and apprehension about the outcome of the pregnancy may best describe the feelings of expectant parents during the second month. Moodiness—from joy to fear to irritability—and fatigue are typical. Focusing on how you will care for yourself to protect and enhance your baby's development is essential to this formative month.

The Growing Baby

What a dramatic month this is in the development of your baby! Significant transformations are occurring. By the end of this second month, your baby has changed from an embyro to a fetus. Why the change in terminology? The baby is no longer just life but also form. All of the parts needed for life have formed. Your baby is starting to look like a miniature human being. Its body structure is set.

Pray for the formation of your baby's body:

Dear God, our Father,

We honor and respect You with the highest regard. Your creative work in our lives right now is sometimes difficult to imagine. We know that every cell of our growing little baby is life from You.

We thank You for how this tiny life is being formed and ask for Your special blessing on every little part. May our child be wonderfully and perfectly designed. Amen.

Let's look at the details of the formation of the baby's infra-structure, the basis for his or her growth during the rest of the pregnancy. The foundation is being laid for the brain, spinal cord, and nervous system from an outer layer of cells. The brain, more incredible than any computer ever built, is developing at a phenomenal rate and growing to fill the baby's head.

Say a prayer for your baby's mind, in your own words or in these I have written for you:

Our baby's mind, dear God, we commit to You. The amazing role that all those millions of neurons will play in the growth and development of our child is beyond our comprehension. Safeguard his brain and nervous system not only as it now is

forming but during the rest of this pregnancy and throughout his life. May You bless him with a quick and healthy
mind that he will use to honor You. With love and trust in
Your unlimited power, we praise You. Amen.

The other internal organs are forming from the middle and
inner layers of cells. The embryonic heart and lungs are completely developed by the end of this month. Taste and tooth
buds are forming. The digestive tract is taking form. The optic
vesicles form the basis for future eyesight.

External features develop, making the baby look more
human. Even though the eyelids fuse over the newly formed
eyes and remain closed for several months, the facial features are
assuming a definite shape, with indentations for ears and nose
forming on the sides of the head and in the center of the face.
Limbs are beginning to show distinctive divisions into arms,
elbows, forearms, hands, thighs, knees, lower legs, and feet. The
long "bones," made of cartilage that will gradually be replaced
by bone cells, are developing. Tiny fingers and toes are beginning to differentiate. Because the baby's back is forming faster
than his front, he is still shaped like a "C."

Your care for your developing baby will be demonstrated by
your discipline in caring for yourself. God cares about your
baby's development and reminds us of the reliability of His care
for us in a mother's care for her child.

Can a woman forget her nursing child,
And have no compassion on the son of her womb?
Even these may forget, but I will not forget you.
Behold I have inscribed you on the palms of My hands.

ISAIAH 49:15-16a, NASB

Changes in the Mother-to-Be

If you have not already become aware of the sacrifice a mother is required to make for her child, you will. The command a baby has over your body increases throughout the pregnancy. Your body is now dedicated and adapting to the growth, development, and nurturing of this baby.

The sacrificial giving of parenting starts with pregnancy. We have to take care of ourselves for the primary purpose of our child's best interests; this relinquishment of our desires for the good of our children is required of us. Christ's gift of Himself to us, His children, empowers us to forfeit our desires and needs for the benefit of our children during pregnancy and parenting.

O Lord, you are never weary of doing me good. Let me never be weary of doing your service. But as you have pleasure in the prosperity of your servants, so let me take pleasure in the service of my Lord, and abound in your work, and in your love and praise evermore. O fill up all that is wanting, reform whatever is amiss in me, perfect the thing that concerns me. Let the witness of your pardoning love ever abide in my heart.

John Wesley[1]

Pray a prayer of self-sacrifice. You may want to use these words I have written for you:

Dear God,

Our prayer is to be Jesus to our child. Give us a sense of deep joy in knowing that our sacrificing for the best of our developing baby is just a token of what You did for us. Bless us as we give ourselves to You and to our child. In Christ's name, Amen.

Your body is starting to change its shape. Even though ideally you should not yet be gaining weight, it is common to lose your waistline as early as the second month. Because of the increase in the hormone progesterone, your bowels may have slowed down a bit, causing bloating. The bowel distention in addition to the swelling of the uterus will affect your figure. To reduce bowel sluggishness, drink eight to ten glasses of water a day and get your quota of fiber in your diet.

Fatigue and sleepiness often increase in the second month because so much energy is needed from your body to promote the incredible changes that are happening in the baby's development. Your nap is a must by now!

Many of the symptoms of the first month continue during this month. Frequent urination may be reduced at night if you drink more fluid during the day and less during the evening. Drink constantly during the day if you're going to cut back for the night. Increased breast tenderness can be soothed with a supportive, well-fitting bra. Sexual play may need to be adjusted so as not to irritate your breasts. Talk to your husband. Direct him in the kind of touch that feels good, and guide him away from irritating touch. You may have nasal stuffiness because of the increased estrogen levels. A cool air vaporizer is often helpful; just remember not to use any nasal sprays or decongestants because of the danger they may pose to the developing baby. If you have specific questions about what is safe and what is not, ask your physician. You will do well, especially during these early months of pregnancy, to err on the side of caution.

Pray a prayer of giving yourself to God, and He will fill you with His strength:

Take, Lord, and receive all my liberty,
My memory, my understanding, and my entire will—
All that I have and call my own.
You have given it all to me.
To you, Lord, I return it.
Everything is yours; do with it what you will.
Give me only your love and your grace.
That's enough for me.

St. Ignatius of Loyola[2]

Decision of the Month

How Will You Care for Yourself for Baby's Sake?

The tasks of this month will coordinate with this decision. The basis for the decision is in the chapter "On Pregnancy." But before you attempt to apply those recommendations, take some time to understand yourself and what is likely to work for you.

In the past, when you have had to make changes in your lifestyle, what has encouraged you in those transitions? Has it helped to write out a plan, to rely on a friend or your spouse, to build in a reward system, to pray about it, to have a checklist, or to really understand why you are doing what you are doing and review your reasons regularly? Envision yourself with your baby. The reality of creating a new life is often the strongest motivating factor. Change is difficult. Pregnancy and parenting require change.

The decision to care for yourself encompasses many choices:

- How will you handle nutrition?
- How will you ensure adequate rest?
- How will you keep physically fit and prepare your body for labor and delivery?

- Have you been diligent in eliminating any intake that could harm your baby?
- Can you reduce stress?

Pray for positive decision-making and discipline in keeping those decisions to nurture and protect. Pray in your own words, or use these words written for you:

Dear Heavenly Father,
Even as You have blessed us with this new life, give us wisdom to make the correct decisions and discipline to practice what we believe. You know what is best for our baby's growth and development. Forgive us when we fail, and protect our baby from our mistakes. We thank You. Amen.

Tasks, Hopes, and Dreams for the Month

Make a Plan for Taking Care of Yourself
I'm beginning to sound repetitious—and intentionally so. Once you've made your decisions about caring for yourself in ways that are best for your growing family, those decisions have to be transferred into action.

Eating plan: Many factors will influence the actual accomplishment of your goals regarding good nutrition and the elimination of harmful substances from your diet. If you have a history of dieting, you will probably have baggage associated with making an eating plan. Shifting your attitude from one of restriction to one of ensuring adequate intake of nutrients will help you. For example, protein intake has been emphasized. Why is that so important? The development of the baby's brain cells is particularly dependent upon available protein; soy beans contain all the essential amino acids to help your body synthesize protein. So this month, when the baby's brain is growing so fast, you may want to include a daily shake with pure soy powder, yogurt, milk, and fruit.

Don't look at your eating plan as a diet. The purpose of any restrictions you face while pregnant is threefold: to protect the baby, to avoid substitution of nonessential food or drink for nutrients essential for the baby's growth, and to eliminate uncomfortable symptoms and health complications for you.

We've talked about the first two purposes in the chapter "On Pregnancy." To help with the third, here are specific dietary adjustments that may help relieve specific symptoms.

For fluid retention (swelling) or high blood pressure: reduce salt, eat asparagus, and drink extra water. For fatigue: increase proteins and vegetables, take your prenatal vitamin, and get extra sleep. For cramps (uterine, leg, eye twitches): Take a prenatal vitamin that has adequate magnesium and calcium in proportion to phosphorus and follow the suggested eating plan. For constipation: Take in adequate fiber, drink lots of fluid (warm water with lemon or prune juice upon awakening), and exercise. For blood sugar swings (cravings, moodiness): reduce simple carbohydrates (making sure you continue to get your three to five servings of whole grains and legumes), eliminate sugar and white flour, and eat small amounts of protein six times a day.

Plan for Rest: How many hours of sleep are you getting every twenty-four hours? Are you still feeling sleepy or experiencing fatigue? Can you increase your nighttime sleep? What about taking a thirty-minute nap at your sleepiest time of the day? If you don't see yourself as a napper, try resting and setting an electronic timer for the designated amount of time each day, at about the same time of day.

Exercise plan: What type of exercise have you been used to? Does that need to change because it is too strenuous or jarring for pregnancy? Do you live in a high-altitude area? Talk to your health care professional about adapting your exercise to the altitude so you do not interfere with an adequate supply of oxygen to the baby. Set realistic goals for exercise so you can be successful. If you find yourself falling short of your goals, readjust them to make them manageable. Choose activities for your plan that are the most enjoyable of all possible choices.

Elimination plan: Take a day to attend to every single thing you put on your skin or into your body or breathe in. Is there anything you are using that could be detrimental?[3]

If you are having difficulty giving up something like caffeine, seek encouragement from someone who will be your ally yet hold you accountable. Also, work into your plan some form of reward. Your reward may be an intentional deviation from your plan by eating something that may not be ideal but won't harm your baby.

Stress reduction plan: When we enjoy what we do, take care of our needs for sleep and nutrition, and are not taking in chemicals that stress our bodies, hard work can be great. However, if work produces emotional or physical stress, then changing or reducing certain activities and responsibilities that place demands on your body may be a necessary decision to consider this month. Talk about this decision and make a plan with your spouse.

Prayers and Scripture

Because of your unfailing love, I can enter your house; with deepest awe I will worship at your Temple. Lead me in the right path, O Lord.... Tell me clearly what to do, and show me which way to turn.

PSALM 5:7-8, NLT

God, you will keep in perfect peace those whose minds are fixed on you; for in returning and rest we shall be saved; in quietness and trust shall be our strength.

ISAIAH 26:3; 30:15[4]

Bless the Lord, who is my rock.
  He gives me strength....
He is my loving ally and my fortress,
  my tower of safety, my deliverer.
He stands before me as a shield, and I take refuge in him.
  PSALM 144:1-2, NLT

The Third Month:
Nourishing and Cherishing

Transition is the key word to describe this month. The baby's development is shifting from formation to growth. The mother's body is adapting to the changes of pregnancy. As a couple, you will find your thinking shifting from an emphasis on being pregnant to the reality that being pregnant means you are going to be parents. The decision of this month (and your decisions for the rest of your lives) will now consider what is best for your child and how that perspective can be balanced with your personal wishes and needs. Your dreams and hopes for your baby, and for you as a family, are becoming specific and real.

The Growing Baby

The first two months were loaded with daily changes. Now the process of formation slows, and growth becomes the primary activity of the last seven months. As one author stated, "If the whole course of pregnancy were fitted into a single nine-to-five working day, all the important development in the fetus would have taken place by the midmorning coffee break."[1]

By the end of the third month, the membranes that make up the amniotic sac containing the fluid in which the baby floats have completely formed. The internal organs, though very tiny, are all present and functioning. The baby's head accounts for half of his or her body length, since the brain developed so quickly during the past month. Muscles and bones are growing quickly. The body will grow rapidly from this time on and will assume a less C-shaped, more upright posture.

There are some formative refinements taking place. Arms, hands, fingers, legs, feet, and toes are becoming distinct. The ears form completely during this month. The iris, the colored part of the eye, develops, though the baby's true eye color will not be determined until several weeks or more after birth. Vocal cords form.

The baby's activities indicate uncontrolled muscle functioning. There are involuntary twitches, swallowing and sucking motions, and opening and closing of the mouth. The baby begins to secrete urine, which is sterile and is swallowed with the amniotic fluid or excreted into the mother's circulatory system. Soon the baby will be making most of the amniotic fluid himself from what he squirts out of his urinary system.

The sex of the child, which was determined at conception, is becoming differentiated. The ultrasound will not detect the sex of the baby until sometime in the next two months, however.

> So God created people in his own image;
>   God patterned them after himself;
>   male and female he created them.

GENESIS 1:27, NLT

Say a prayer for the sexuality of your child. Pray in your own words or use these words written for you:

Heavenly Father,

How pleased we are that You designed us as men and women, boys and girls. We thank You for the gender of our little one. Prepare us for that gender. Help us to protect, nurture, and develop the sexuality of our child right from the moment of birth. Keep our child from painful sexual encounters. Give affirmation of sexual feelings and direction and strength for sexual choices throughout our child's life. Amen.

Your baby's individual characteristics and behaviors will become distinct and he or she will look clearly human by the end of the third month. The specifics vary from baby to baby, following inherited patterns.

Say a prayer of praise for your child's individuality:

For the uniqueness of this little person we thank You, Lord. We pray that we will be consistent in affirming Your design of our child. Amen.

Changes in the Mother-to-Be

"Will I ever again have energy?" may be your most prominent wonderment. "I'm exhausted beyond belief!" You are likely to continue to feel more tired than usual throughout this month.

Now might be a good time to say a prayer of thanks and recognition of the source of your strength. You may want to use your own words, or these words written for you:

Dear God,

I know You care about me even as You have told us that You care about the birds and the grass. There are times I feel so tired. I need an extra boost of Your strength. Help me to use my energy and time wisely and to take care of myself. Thank You for this very special time in our family's life. Amen.

Your appetite may increase as the baby has new demands for nourishment that cause you to burn calories faster. This increase in metabolism may also increase perspiration and warmth in your body. Your body will need more fluid, so this is a reminder to keep that glass or bottle of water with you and keep sipping throughout the day. Use your increased hunger to make certain you are getting your four servings of calcium per day. Yogurt, milk, cheese, broccoli, salmon, and sardines are all great sources of calcium, which is so essential to the rapid growth of the baby's muscles and bones during this month and throughout the rest of the pregnancy. Just a reminder: avoid refined sugar as much as possible. Sugar contributes nothing to a healthy pregnancy. Grabbing for sweets when you are hungry will not help your baby's growth and certainly will not promote your health or energy. An apple is a good source of vitamins and minerals and will give you that quick boost of energy you may be craving.

You satisfy me more than the richest of foods.

PSALM 63:5, NLT

Set a guard, O Lord, over my mouth; keep watch over the door of my lips ... and do not let me eat of their delicacies.

PSALM 141:3-4, NASB

If your shape didn't change last month, it certainly will during this time, because your uterus will grow to about the size of a grapefruit. It is now too big to sit in your pelvis and will move up into your abdomen, so that your waist will no longer fit within your regular clothing. You will start to gain weight, about two to three pounds during this month.

Lightheadedness, dizziness, and headaches may be the result of hormonal changes and increased need for blood supply for you and the baby. Make sure you are getting enough iron. Prune juice or dried prunes are not only a good source of iron but also will help relieve any tendency toward constipation. If constipation is interfering right now, increase your fluid, vegetable, fruit, and whole grain (wheat, rice, or oat bran) intake and your aerobic exercise. Allow yourself a consistent daily time for bowel movements.

As you move to the end of this third month, you are completing the first third, or trimester, of your pregnancy. Your body and feelings will be adjusting to the demands and changes of pregnancy and you will be moving into a more energetic and serene stage—the second trimester.

Decision of the Month

Do You Want to Know the Sex of Your Baby?

This is a decision new to this generation. My husband and I had no option to know. With more advanced technology and increases in knowledge come additional choices and responsibilities.

To know or not to know is a matter of personal preference. Independent of your spouse, think through whether you would like to know and why or why not. You might even want to write down your thoughts before you discuss the issue with your spouse. Read your spouse's thoughts, reflect on them, and rephrase for your spouse what you sense he or she feels about this choice and why. Even if you don't agree, you will feel less tension about your differences if you understand each other's views.

Why choose not to be told the gender of your baby? The most common reason is because you want the surprise at the moment of birth. The more serious concern, however, is that the professional reading the ultrasound could make an error. Ask for the percentage of certainty.

My bias is that the advantages of knowing your baby's gender outweigh not knowing. There is increasing evidence that experiences in the womb affect the child. Knowing and affirming your unborn baby's sex will, I suspec, have long-term benefits for your child's gender identity and self-acceptance.

Say a prayer for guidance in your gender identification decision.

Dear Heavenly Father,

You formed and designed our baby to be a boy or a girl. Even though we come to this pregnancy with our wishes, we *do* want Your will to be done here on earth as it is in heaven. In the case of our baby's gender, we know Your will is the right choice. In a world of so much information and so many choices, decisions have become more difficult. Give us wisdom as we approach this decision of knowing or not knowing what You already know—the sex of our baby. Help us as a couple to care about each other's feelings so that we can come to the decision with love and respect. Be with the doctor who interprets the ultrasound. In Jesus' name, Amen.

Tasks, Hopes, and Dreams for the Month

Plan for the Spiritual Formation of Your Child

The spiritual formation of your child needs to be deliberately promoted rather than assumed. You can decide how you as a family will want to incorporate spiritual development into your lifestyle by referring back to that section near the end of the parenting chapter. You will also want to consider how your parents imparted or taught you about faith and values, and how your relationship with God developed. How does your church encourage spiritual formation for children? Age-appropriate books, tapes, and videos can provide teaching opportunities. Praying with children can be a precious time of hearing their hearts.

O God, make the door of this house wide enough to receive all who need human love and fellowship; narrow enough to shut out all envy, pride, and strife.

Make its threshold smooth enough to be no stumbling block to children nor to straying feet, but rugged and strong enough to turn back the tempter's power. God, make the door of this house the gateway to thine eternal kingdom.

On St. Stephen's Wallbrook, London[2]

Prayers and Scripture

Dear God,

Help me to teach my child that if we admit our sins, You will forgive our sins and wipe away all evidence of wrongdoing (adapted from 1 John 1:9).

Dear God,

I pray that my child will grow as Jesus matured, growing up in both body and spirit, blessed by both God and people (adapted from Luke 2:52).

I will teach my child about God when we sit in the house and when we go for walks and when we go to bed and when we get up in the morning (adapted from Deuteronomy 6:7).

Help us to teach our child to fill his mind with things that are true, noble, reputable, authentic, compelling, gracious—things to praise, not things to curse. Help him to put into practice what he has learned from us (adapted from Philippians 4:8).

Lord, I pray for the child I am carrying in my womb. Even from this early stage, may this baby feel my love and acceptance. Oh, the dreams and plans I have for him or her! But, Lord, help me to be willing to lay them aside for Your greater purposes. I'm trusting You, Lord, to help me carry this child full-term and have a safe delivery. Be with all the doctors and nurses who will be attending me. Give them wisdom beyond their experience during the birth of my baby. Thank you, Lord, for giving life! Amen.[3]

We have this moment to hold in our hands
And to touch as it slips through our fingers like sand.
Yesterday's gone and tomorrow may never come,
But we have this moment today.[1]

The Fourth Month: Settling In

Settling in. Growing. Maturing. These are the words that best describe the beginning of the second trimester. The baby's primary functions at this stage are growth, maturation, and increased responsiveness. You as a couple are likely to focus on the need for wardrobe adjustments for the mother-to-be; living situation adjustments for your growing family; the transition into parenthood or additional children; and increased interaction with your responsive unborn baby.

The Growing Baby

During this month, the baby's growth is remarkable. His body is catching up with his head, and he is beginning to be proportioned more like a newborn. The baby's organs are maturing, and his abdomen is now large enough to contain his intestines.

87

His muscles are stronger, so that he can hold his head erect, squint, yawn, stretch, make a fist, make faces, and suck his thumb. Even the nails on his toes and fingers are forming.

Say a prayer for the physical development of your baby. Pray these words written for you or use your own words:

We thank You, God, for all the little parts of our baby's body that You have made to work in this intricate form. We ask that our baby grow in strength and maturity. We entrust our unborn baby's body to You. Amen.

Because of the sensory functions that are developing in your baby, this month marks the beginning of her connection with you. She now can hear you even though she cannot yet hear voices outside of your body. The amniotic fluid is a great conductor of sound, which means your heartbeat, digestive processes, and voice are resonant to her. The baby responds to her lips being stroked by sucking. She moves her hands over her eyes to shield them when a bright light is shined on your abdomen.

Pray for connection with your child and your ability to listen to him or her.

Dear Father,

You listen to our prayers and hear us when we come to You. May we do the same with our children. Teach us to be more like You. Amen.

You may feel the baby move sometime this month or next. Even though he has been moving since the seventh week, his small size and weak muscles have not allowed the movements to be strong enough for you to actually feel them. At first you may be unsure whether what you have felt was the baby or just something going on inside of you. Many women do not notice fetal movement until at least the twentieth week, which would be near the beginning of next month.

Say a prayer of praise for the gift of life, and pray for the spiritual life of your child. Use your own words or these words written for you:

Heavenly Father,

You are the giver of life here on earth and eternally. You promise us fullness of life through trust in You. You have proven Your unconditional love toward us. We pray that our child will grow to know and receive Your love. Even now, Lord, may Your Spirit bless our child. Thank You for Your gift of Yourself to us. In Jesus' name, Amen.

Your baby's thin skin is covered with a fine, downlike layer of hair, but her blood vessels can still be seen through the skin and hair because there is no fat under the skin. Soon deposits of brown fat will form to generate heat until shortly after birth. The baby's circulatory system is working. Her heart is pumping the blood just as it will after birth. Bones are hardening.

During this month, the baby's external sex organs become distinctly male or female. At the very end of this month or the beginning of the fifth month, the genitals can be identified on ultrasound, but usually the ultrasound isn't done until a few weeks later, around the twentieth week. By about this same time, a little girl's ovaries contain all of the millions of eggs that will be available for reproduction when she is an adult.

Take a good look at God's wonders—
they'll take your breath away.

PSALM 66:5, THE MESSAGE

Changes in the Mother-to-Be

Starting your second trimester can be a big relief. If you struggled during the first three months, you are likely noticing a positive change. Nausea is lessened or absent. You are probably getting some of your old energy back. And you aren't urinating as frequently, since the uterus has shifted up and away from the bladder. The middle trimester is often the best of the three because the early hormonal symptoms gradually dissipate and the encumbrance of a huge abdomen is not yet a burden.

Say a prayer of praise:

Dear God,
Thank you! Everything in me says, "Thank you!"
  Angels listen as I sing my thanks.
I kneel in worship facing your holy temple
  and say it again: "Thank you!"
Thank you for your love,
  thank you for your faithfulness;
Most holy is your name,
  most holy is your Word.
The moment I called out, you stepped in;
  you made my life large with strength.

PSALM 138:1-2, THE MESSAGE

The primary symptoms during this middle stage of pregnancy have to do with increased blood volume. Your veins may be more pronounced. Wearing supportive tights or nylon stockings may be helpful for the veins in your legs. Varicose veins in your rectum—hemorrhoids—can result from the increased blood volume and constipation. Exercise, fiber, and fluids are essential to prevention and relief. Your gums may bleed more easily. Make sure to maintain your regular regimen for dental examinations and cleanings, gum stimulation, flossing and brushing your teeth. You may have nasal stuffiness or nose-bleeds. Keeping your nasal passages moist may help.

Life is changing. Changes can be exciting, but they also involve giving up freedom, sleep, time, and many other valuable commodities. Feelings of ambivalence associated with becoming parents for the first time or again may revisit you. If you are someone who was given to freely by your parents, these changes may be easy. If you had to do the giving in your home as a child, you may feel resentment or you may look forward to reversing the pattern of your parents. You still have time to deal with difficult feelings about becoming a parent before the baby comes. Talking with someone close to you may help you understand and work through your negative feelings so that you don't pass on to your child the errors of the parenting you received. If not, seek the help of a professional therapist. Everyone will benefit!

Pray this prayer written for you:

Dear God, our Father,

At this time of change, Your unchangeableness is a comfort. You not only give us strength, You also provide a sense of stability. I am so blessed to know that You are the same yesterday, today, and forever. Amen.

I love Thee, O Lord, my strength.
The Lord is my rock and my fortress and my deliverer,
My God, my rock, in whom I take refuge.

PSALM 18:1-2a, NASB

What a thrill to know that your baby hears and reacts to your tone of voice. Not having had this knowledge, I have enjoyed witnessing the amazing connection between our two grandbabies and their parents that started before birth and was evidenced immediately at birth.

Sex may have been put on the back burner during the first trimester because of cramping or spotting, fatigue, sensitive breasts, or nausea, yet sex can be enjoyed throughout pregnancy unless complications warrant restrictions. During the last three months, the logistics of sex may limit your activity. This midtrimester is the time to go for it.

Sex will be different when you are pregnant. The change in sensations can be fun and add newness to your experience. Sometimes when women switch into their "being a mother" role, they no longer think of themselves as sexual partners. Do remember that your children will come and go, but you will always be a sexual person, long after they are out on their own. Physically and emotionally, the benefits of sex during pregnancy far outweigh any hesitancy you might have. The process your body goes through during a sexual response is very helpful for the circulation and preparation of your genitals for childbirth.

God designed sex for three purposes: unity, pleasure, and procreation. The procreation function has been accomplished for now. This is the time to focus on closeness and unity as well as your body's pleasure.

Decision of the Month

Breastfeed or Bottle?
This is an important decision. You will want to gather information about breastfeeding and weigh the factors of your situation in order to make the best decision about feeding your baby. In

some cases this may be not so much a decision as a given. You may know you will not be able to breastfeed, or you may just know you will.

Medical issues can interfere with breastfeeding. We had a friend who, even with the best help from lactation specialists, found that her nipples just couldn't handle the sucking. She pumped and gave her baby her breast milk by bottle, which was a great solution. Others have had breast surgery that interrupts the milk flow of the breasts. You may have an illness or carry an infection that could be transmitted to the baby. You may need medication that would be harmful to the baby when transmitted through your milk. Your baby may have difficulty sucking. If you wish to breastfeed and cannot, you will grieve that loss.

What Are the Advantages of Breastfeeding?

- Your breasts are always available and ready.
- Breastfeeding is economical.
- Bonding is facilitated. The hormone prolactin is believed to increase motherly attachment.
- The uterus contracts during breastfeeding, reducing hemorrhaging after childbirth and more quickly helping the uterus return to its prepregnancy size.
- The mother can eat more than she is used to and lose her pregnancy weight.
- Breastfeeding promotes rest and relaxation without concern about how much milk is left in the bottle or if the baby is getting air or choking. Plan to *allow an hour* for each feeding *or ignore the time*. Even though the basic needs are met after about ten minutes on each breast, the more nutritious milk is produced while the baby continues to nurse.

- Breast sucking is stronger than bottle sucking and promotes correct palate formation.
- Allergic reactions will be delayed or reduced.
- Lower incidence of SIDS (Sudden Infant Death Syndrome) is reported in babies who are breastfed for at least the first four months.[2]
- Breastfed babies are shown to be less likely to struggle with obesity later in life. One study showed that the longer the baby was breastfed with no introduction of solid foods, the less likely the child was to be obese later.[3] The fat content of breast milk changes according to the needs of the baby when the mother is getting sufficient nutrition. Hence, there is less likelihood of overfeeding.
- Breast milk has more nutrients, has a healthier balance of minerals, and is more digestible than formula.
- The greatest benefit of breastfeeding or giving breast milk by bottle is the continued immunity it provides the baby.

Why You Might Choose to Bottle-feed.
- Perhaps your mother did and recommends it.
- Maybe your friends have bottle-fed their babies.
- You may feel intimidated or uncertain of your ability to breastfeed. Breastfeeding is not an innate skill; it has to be learned.
- You may have to go back to work. (With a breast pump, you can collect and freeze bottles of breast milk.)
- Your husband might have difficulty sharing your breasts with the baby.
- Your physician may promote bottle-feeding.
- The intimate connection inherent in breastfeeding may make you uncomfortable.

Once your decision is clear, you can move ahead with preparing for either breast- or bottle-feeding. Even if you will be breastfeeding, you will want to purchase some bottles and nipples for water or pumped breast milk. Choose a variety of nipples. You may have to try several before you find the one your baby will take. Do the same with pacifiers. If you are planning to bottle-feed, study the various formulas. Attend to the ingredients.

Should you be undecided, give breastfeeding a try. You can always stop, but starting to breastfeed after some time has passed since birth can be difficult, if not impossible. Breastfeeding even for a few weeks has significant benefit for the baby.

You brought me safely from my mother's womb and led me to trust you when I was a nursing infant.

PSALM 22:9, NLT

Rejoice…. Drink deeply of her glory even as an infant drinks at its mother's generous breasts. Her children will be nursed at her breasts, carried in her arms, and treated with love. I will comfort you as a child is comforted by its mother.

ISAIAH 66:10-13, NLT

Tasks, Hopes, and Dreams for the Month

Developing a Birthing Plan
Start by reading as much as you can find in books or on the Internet and applying what you have learned in childbirth classes. Talk to your physician or midwife about issues and

choices to consider for birthing. Then brainstorm as a couple and jot down your ideas as they come to you. Think through all your ideas about how you want to give birth. Make a list of what you consider important to your birthing process. Take that list to your next appointment with your practitioner. If you want a more formal plan or want more input regarding your choices, *Pregnancy Week-by-Week*[4] by Dr. Jane MacDougall has an excellent form for you to complete.

Pray for motivation and wisdom in making your birthing plan. Pray for the correct guidance from your practitioner and other resources. Pray for release from unnecessary and unwarranted fears.

Father, may Your will be done in our process of giving birth. Help us to have the diligence, wisdom, and courage to do our part to prepare for this life-changing event. Release us from fears. We put our trust in You. In Jesus' name, Amen.

Selecting Birthing Preparation Instruction

Childbirth education and preparation is designed to help women cope with childbirth through active participation and increased decision-making. The preparation makes childbirth a more rewarding experience for the mother, her husband, and the entire family.

The best-known methods available today are Lamaze (202-857-1128), Modified Lamaze, Bradley (818-788-6662; Box 5224, Sherman Oaks, CA 91413-5224), Dick-Read (415-456-3143), and Gamper (312-248-8100). These all have many common ingredients and vary depending on the particular instructor. You might surf the Internet to get as much information as you can on these or other childbirth preparation opportunities. You can also contact the International Childbirth Education Association at 612-854-8660. The success of all of the training programs is the consistency with which you train and the involvement of your coach during actual labor and delivery.

I somtimes wonder if because epidurals (a type of regional anesthesia used to relieve pain during labor and delivery) are so freely used during labor, the motivation for advance preparation is reduced. I am convinced that the best combination is to prepare as though an epidural will not be available and then use the epidural as needed. I suspect labor and delivery is longer and harder for those who have not diligently and consistently practiced the exercises and do not have the benefit of a confident coach.

Selecting Infant and Child Care Classes
The hospital or birthing center where you will be delivering will probably offer infant and child care instruction as well as CPR and breastfeeding classes. The American Red Cross and your local YWCA may be other resources. Before the class starts, determine its content and the teaching methods to be used, so you will not be disappointed. The more you prepare, the better.

Prayer and Scripture

My child, listen to me and treasure my instructions. Tune your ears to wisdom, and concentrate on understanding. Cry out for insight and understanding. Search for them as you would for lost money or hidden treasure. Then you will understand what is right, just, and fair, and you will know how to find the right course of action every time.

PROVERBS 2:1-3,9, NLT

Dear God,

We thank You for Your promise that You have "not given us a spirit of fear and timidity, but of power, love and self-discipline" (2 Timothy 1:7, NLT). Amen.

Meanwhile, the moment we get tired in the waiting, God's Spirit is right alongside helping us along. If we don't know how or what to pray, it doesn't matter. He does our praying in and for us, making prayer out of our wordless sighs, our aching groans. He knows us far better than we know ourselves, knows our pregnant condition, and keeps us present before God. That is why we can be so sure that every detail of our lives of love for God is worked into something good.

ROMANS 8:26-28, THE MESSAGE

The Fifth Month: Experiencing Life

The theme of this month is *life!* The baby is letting you know he is alive, and you have so much happening in your life as well. The middle of this month marks the halfway point of your pregnancy. The baby's structure is set now, so much is beginning to awaken. Similar to the construction of a home, the structure is built and now every detail is filled in with all the color and softness that makes the building a home.

The Growing Baby

The excitement of the fifth month is that the movement of the baby—the "quickening"—will be clearly evident to the mother. By now the baby is big enough and strong enough to make himself known. His bones are harder, and his muscles are strengthening every week; his more sophisticated movements evidence this. His kicking, punching, and tumbling in the amniotic sac will be evident to Mommy from now.

Say a prayer of praise for the life of your unborn child:

Heavenly Father,
   You are the giver and sustainer of life. What a joy it is to feel this precious little one kicking. Thank You for this baby's life. Amen.

Not only is the baby moving, but she is also able to hear sounds outside the mother's body. The whole family can talk and sing to the baby. You need to be aware of your tone of voice around the baby. Loud sounds will startle her or cause her to raise her arms to cover her ears. Rock and roll music has been shown to cause agitated movements. On the contrary, calming music played near the mother's abdomen during pregnancy can be used after birth to calm a fussy baby. Classical music, hymns, or soft, harmonious popular tunes produce tranquillity.

Say a prayer for the connection of all family members with the new baby:

Dear Lord,

In our excitement about this new baby we also need sensitivity and care for our other children's reactions to this baby coming into their world. Show us ways to involve them with the baby. Give us generous and unconditional love for each of them. Give us energy to go that extra mile in meeting their needs, so that when the baby comes they will be deeply secure. In Jesus' name, Amen.

The baby's internal organs are maturing at an astonishing speed, but the lungs are still insufficiently developed to cope with conditions outside the uterus. Early in this month, somewhere between the eighteenth and the twentieth weeks, the doctor can hear the heartbeat with a stethoscope. You will probably get to listen, too. The ultrasound is usually done around the same time. This is the time when the sex of your child can be determined.

The development of the brain of the unborn child is a magical phenomenon. Trillions of brain cells are multiplying wildly and forming purposeful electrical connections between various parts of the brain. The electrical activity of these brain cells actually affects the structure of the brain and the explosion of learning that occurs after birth. This month of pregnancy begins the next five to six years of significant brain growth. Even though there are varying opinions on whether playing music for and talking to your baby now will really enchance brain cell growth, stimulating input will certainly promote parent-child bonding. Research does confirm that sensory experiences after birth trigger electrical activity that enhances brain growth.

Pray for the development of your baby's mind. Use your own words, or these written for you:

Our Father,

We are in awe of the miracle of Your creation of our baby's mind. Protect his mind now and after birth. Help us to interact with our child in healthy, nurturing ways that will promote his potential and our relationship with him without pressuring him. Give him wisdom as he matures. Thank You, God. Amen.

If the Holy Spirit controls your mind, there is life and peace.

ROMANS 8:6, NLT

Don't copy the behavior and customs of this world, but let God transform you into a new person by changing the way you think. Then you will know what God wants you to do, and you will know how good and pleasing and perfect his will really is.

ROMANS 12:2, NLT

My children, listen to me. Listen to your father's instruction. Pay attention and grow wise.... Learn to be wise, and develop good judgment. Getting wisdom is the most important thing you can do! And whatever else you do, get good judgment.

PROVERBS 4:1, 5, 7, NLT

Body growth slows now. The baby is half the length she will be at birth. She starts putting on weight quickly to catch up with her length.

As the months of the pregnancy progress, the growing baby's uniqueness becomes more and more pronounced. The hair on his head begins to grow. She may accidentally suck her thumb as her sucking skills develop and her hand happens to find her mouth. Facial features, expressions, movements, and responses unique to her are becoming more obvious. Your baby's facial expressions, determined by muscle alignment, already reflect your families'. The baby establishes his rhythmic sleep and awake pattern, similar to what he will follow after birth. Sleep positions are also particular to individual babies. Both of our grandsons positioned their heads back to fall asleep. Both were in the posterior position before birth, so may have learned while in the womb to sleep with their necks extended.

Your task as parents is to get to know your child as a one-of-a-kind creation entrusted to you to nurture and to maximize his potential.

Pray this prayer for the unique development of your child:

Dear God,

Christ taught that You care so much about each person that You even know the number of hairs on our heads. The psalmist writes: "Like an open book, you watched me grow from conception to birth" (Psalm 139:16, THE MESSAGE). You know every nuance of our baby's physical characteristics. Help us to love every detail of his body and his person, even as You so love us. In Jesus' name, Amen.

Changes in the Mother-to-Be

Feeling the movements of your baby is a comfort even though the baby's activity may interrupt your sleep and tire you. Most of the changes you experience from this point on are the result of the baby getting heavier. The increased weight of the baby will put additional pressure on your back and pelvis. Lower abdominal discomfort is usually the result of the stretching of the ligaments that support the uterus. If the pain should become intense, be sure to contact your practitioner. You have probably just strained a muscle or ligament, but you should be checked.

There are precautions you can take to reduce discomforts and complications. Ask your health care practitioner for a list of tips to avoid backaches. The changes your body is making in preparation for childbirth as well as the shift in your body's balance because of your protruding abdomen may cause discomfort.

Pregnancy raises body temperature and increases blood flow to the skin, causing the "glow" of pregnancy. Around the middle of pregnancy, however, certain skin changes can be a nuisance. Spidery-looking veins may appear on your upper body. The "mask" of pregnancy, a darkening of the pigment of the skin on the upper cheekbones, is exaggerated by exposure to the sun. Women with darker complexions are more susceptible. A woman may get a dark line on her abdomen that goes from her umbilicus (belly button) to her pubic hair. Other women develop red itchiness on their palms or the soles of their feet. Still others get an itchy pregnancy rash. All symptoms should be reported to your physician.

As your baby gains weight quickly during this month, you will need to eat when you are hungry. Choose foods that will give you energy, nourish the baby, and not exaggerate any symptoms you might be having. Cravings are common and sometimes rather unusual. Be certain you are getting a balance of the food groups recommended. Take your prenatal vitamin-mineral supplement regularly, and avoid foods of little nutritional value.

Decision of the Month

Knowing the Sex of the Baby, Revisited

If both you and your spouse have not come to peace with each other's views as to knowing or not knowing the sex of your baby, you have several options. You can have the health professional who reads your ultrasound write the sex and his or her certainty about it on a piece of paper and put it into a sealed envelope until you decide. The person most hesitant about knowing should take responsibility for the envelope.

Another option is for the one of you who wishes to know to get the information without sharing it. We have known two couples who did this. In both situations the woman was given the sex identification information at the time of the ultrasound. Each told absolutely no one.

Should you both want to wait to know the gender until birth, be extremely attentive to interacting with the baby. Be careful not to picture or communicate a bias toward one sex or the other.

Tasks, Hopes, and Dreams for the Month

Maximize Your Baby's Potential

There is a fine line between providing your baby with stimulation that can bring out and develop his or her abilities and trying to produce a superkid. The latter is destructive and goal-oriented, often done to make the parents look good. The former is responsibly acting upon the information now available and behaving as good stewards of the talents God has given your child.

There is now a wealth of research implying that we can enhance brain development. Cliff and I did not have the benefit of much of this new research, but we applied what we knew to developing the talents of our children and have experienced the return on our investment.

Some of the stimulation we provided was unintentional. We played "Mozart's Greatest Hits" every night to help our youngest child fall asleep, from the time she was an infant until she was eight or nine years old. It was only later that we heard that Mozart's music might be especially conducive to brain enhancement.

To maximize your child's potential right now and during the next five years while his or her brain is working overtime, I would recommend you get and study the article "How a Child's Brain Develops" (cover title) or "Fertile Minds" (inside title) in the February 3, 1997, issue of *Time* magazine. You can find it at a library or on the Internet (www.Time.com).

Music is a source of stimulation that is vital to brain development. When our youngest daughter was one of twelve students chosen for her high school math team, we were interested to note that ten of the twelve were also violinists.

Pray for wisdom and good judgment in the development of your child's talents.

Dear Father,

What an awesome responsibility You have given us. Thank You for Your confidence in us. We pray for wisdom and good judgment in doing our part to provide our child with the stimulation and conditions most conducive to developing the talents You have given her. May we not be demanding of her but rather encouraging through our consistent giving of ourselves to her. Thank You for hearing our prayer. Amen.

Prepare All Baby Care Items

If you are planning to purchase a new crib or furniture, you may need to order it now in order to have it in time for the baby's arrival. Pamphlets from the doctor's office and most baby care books will have lists of what you will need for your baby. Many items are essential or very beneficial, yet shortlived in their usefulness. You may be able to find some of these items at a secondhand store or garage sale, or as hand-me-downs from friends and family.

If you have other children, involve them in this process of preparation. If the child loses interest, stop what you are doing and focus on him. Avoid any message or implication that communicates, "You can't use this anymore because we're getting it ready for the baby." You don't want to set up competition or give the sense that the baby is replacing the older child.

Prayers and Scripture

Dear Father,

You have promised that "You will keep in perfect peace all who trust in you, whose thoughts are fixed on you!" (Isaiah 26:3). Lord, we trust You for the care of our children and especially this baby that is such a wonderful new life growing inside the womb. Each child is in Your hands. You are the Giver of this life. We are convinced that You will guard this life. We commit ourselves to teach our child to love and honor You. We will train him tenderly and cherish his unique spirit. May we never stifle his potential with harshness or frustration. We commit ourselves to care for him with discipline that encourages his talents and personality, as well as his love for You. Amen.

Dear God,

Even as Solomon prayed a prayer of dedication for the temple, we pray his prayer as a dedication for the life of our child:

"O Lord, God of Israel, there is no God like you in all of heaven or earth. You keep your promises and show unfailing love to all who obey you and are eager to do your will. Listen to my prayer and my request, O Lord my God. Hear the cry and the prayer that your servant is making to you today. May you watch over this Temple both day and night.... May you always hear the prayers I make toward this place" (1 Kings 8:23, 28-29, NLT). Amen.

If you need wisdom—if you want to know what God wants you to do—ask him, and he will gladly tell you. He will not resent your asking. But when you ask him, be sure that you really expect him to answer, for a doubtful mind is as unsettled as a wave of the sea that is driven and tossed by the wind.

JAMES 1:5-6, NLT

The Sixth Month: Becoming Parents

Preparing to survive in the real world is the baby's task during this month. Your task is to prepare for parenthood. Some women struggle throughout their pregnancy, but many find the sixth month to be a time to enjoy looking pregnant and having more energy.

Are you hurting? Pray. Do you feel great? Sing.

JAMES 5:13, THE MESSAGE

The Growing Baby

Each week during this month, the baby's ability to survive outside the mother's womb is greatly improved. He looks like a wrinkled old man, with loose folds, because his skin is forming faster than the fat that will fill in underneath. The small blood vessels just under his thin skin cause a redness that will fade as fat forms. A protective creamy coating called *vermix* forms a barrier between this delicate skin tissue and the amniotic fluid that surrounds it. The baby's face is pretty much as it will look at birth. The eyelashes are formed. The eyes are blue and will be for several months after birth, until they acquire their permanent color. Your baby now opens and closes his eyes, and fingernails extend to the end of his fingers.

Pray for God's protective Spirit to form around your child for a lifetime.

Dear Heavenly Father,

Right now our baby is protected inside the womb by many layers of tissue, muscle, fluid, and even this special creamy coating. When he is born, there will be no more protection between him and the world. Wrap Your arms around this little person, and send Your Spirit to protect him. Thank You for Your care. In Jesus' name, Amen.

And he will be filled with the Holy Spirit, while yet in his mother's womb.

LUKE 1:15b, NASB

The senses are constantly maturing. Touch matures first. The baby can be observed learning about her body and her surroundings through touch. Videos have captured babies playing with the umbilical cord, touching their toes, and stroking various body parts. By this time, your child can very intentionally put her thumb in her mouth. She is increasingly responsive to stimuli from the outside world, and she now responds to external touch and sound. As she reacts to sound her pulse rate increases, and she will move in rhythm to music. Her hearing and the balance systems of the inner ear are now fully developed.

Pray for sensory development and the baby's inner ear balance mechanism. Pray these words written for you:

Dear God,

We pray right now for the development of our baby's senses. May his hearing be acute, his vision sharp, his tactile sense keen, his taste discerning, his sense of smell accurate, and his balance unswerving. In Jesus' name, Amen.

By the end of the month your baby's brain waves resemble those of a newborn. Her brain can now store and remember the sounds she hears, like her parents' voices or music. You can ease your baby's transition from life in the womb to life outside the womb by talking to her so she will recognize you and by playing music that you will play for her after she is born. I witnessed a baby's memory of voices immediately after our first grandson was born. Our children had talked to him throughout the last months of the pregnancy. Hours after he was born, he turned responsively to each of their voices, yet not to any of the grandparents in the room. At first we wondered if his responses were coincidental, but repetition made it obvious that he knew his parents' voices.

Your baby's internal functions are getting stronger. His heartbeat can be heard by putting an ear on the mother's abdomen. His nostrils are opening, and he is learning to make muscular movements that prepare him to draw air into his lungs at birth. Both boys' and girls' sexual and reproductive development is complete. The immune system is producing white blood cells to fight disease and infection. You may soon be able to feel the rhythmic jerking of his hiccuping as he swallows amniotic fluid, a partial source of his nourishment.

Pray for a strong immune system for your child. Use your own words or these words written for you:

Dear Father,

You have not promised that we will be free of disease or infections or suffering in this world. You *have* promised that You will be with us, caring for us in whatever circumstance we find ourselves. We trust You for strength for our baby and for us, should she have to suffer illness. We ask You to bless our baby with a healthy immune system to fight disease and infection. May we do everything in our knowledge and power to enhance the health she brings to this world. Amen.

And this same God who takes care of me will supply all your needs from his glorious riches, which have been given to us in Christ Jesus.

PHILIPPIANS 4:19, NLT

Changes in the Mother-to-Be

The movements of the baby, which are becoming thumps and bumps, will by the end of the month be noticable to anyone placing a hand on your abdomen. Feeling the baby through your abdomen can be a curious and connecting experience for other children, as well as for the two of you.

You will be growing as your baby grows. By the sixth month, your belly is likely to protrude enough to make the rest of your body look smaller in comparison. You will look obviously pregnant, not just thicker. Your feet and ankles may swell because of the pressure of your uterus on the circulation to your legs and feet. Exercising, elevating your feet, lying down, changing positions frequently, and drinking your quota of water can all help. Keep your doctor informed of swelling or other symptoms.

Numbness and tingling in the hands is common during this stage of pregnancy. There is no real solution to this except to give your hands a break from steady use in your job or at home. Shaking out or stretching your hands may also help.

An itchy abdomen is another annoyance, caused by the stretching and drying of your skin. Creams are available, specifically designed for use on pregnant women's abdomens.

Braxton-Hicks contractions may start during this month. They are harmless, painless tightenings of the uterine muscle in preparation for labor and delivery. Welcome them. They are great practice for your uterus.

Just a little reminder to devote some quality time to taking care of yourself and your marriage. Remember, keeping yourself cared for and your marriage strong is not selfish; it is a gift to your child.

Decision of the Month

Determining a Parenting Style

I hope you have been contemplating this decision and praying for clarity in determining the approaches to child rearing that will work best for you and fulfill Scripture's teachings.

As parents, pray for wisdom. Use your own words or these words written for you:

Dear God,

Your wisdom is available to us. Unfortunately it is easily blurred by the conflicting teachings of experts. Help us to be able to take the information we hear, see, and read and sift what we need for our uniquely designed child. With hope and trust in Jesus' name, Amen.

Talk about your past experiences with parenting. If you have children already, what has been your tendency? How are your friends choosing to parent? What system is your church promoting? What were the philosophies and approaches of the parents of the young adults whom you would want as models for your children? What kind of person are you naturally? What approaches have you used when trying to change something about your spouse? Has your method been successful? What tendencies will you need to keep in check?

Pray this prayer written for you:

Dear God,

You know us so well. You know our baby. You know our weaknesses and strengths. Help us see ourselves as You see us so that we might use who we are to honor You in the parenting of our child. In Jesus' name, Amen.

Tasks, Hopes, and Dreams for the Month

Selecting Parenting Preparation

As mentioned earlier, babies don't come with an operating manual. We go to school to learn our vocation or profession in life; we get an owner's manual and video with a new car; but we somehow think we should just know how to be parents. With parents and extended family members at a distance, on-the-job training is less likely to be possible. Do not expect that you will automatically be a good parent. Listen, learn, read, take classes, and ask for help.

In selecting a parenting class or program or working with a mother mentor, use your discernment. Some input and approaches to parenting can steer you in a wrong direction. Some suggested parenting programs:

- Positive Discipline: brad@empoweringpeople.com;
- Active Parenting: cservice@activeparenting.com;
- Strategic Training for Effective Parenting: agsnet.com;
- Family Wellness: families@familywellness.com.

Say a prayer for your ability to learn to parent. Use these words written for you or pray in your own words:

Our Father in heaven,

How we value Your model to us as parents. We know we can never have Your ever-present, unfailing love, exact awareness of when and when not to respond to our children's requests, and judgment in how best to parent our children, but we ask for discernment. Guide us to the best information. Help us to identify and sort out what we should apply to our approach to parenting and what we should regard with hesitation. Lead us, dear Lord. We are open to Your leading. We come to You with grateful hearts. Amen.

The Book of James offers two teachings that might be helpful in your selection of parenting education and in your actual practice. The first is that we are not to be swayed by the popular or the general public opinion.

> My dear friends, don't let public opinion influence how you live out our glorious, Christ-originated faith.
>
> JAMES 2:1, THE MESSAGE

The second is that we are to be directed in our decisions by listening to God through His Word and then responding with action.

> Don't fool yourself into thinking that you are a listener when you are ... letting the Word go in one ear and out the other. Act on what you hear! Those who hear and don't act are like those who glance in the mirror, walk away, and two minutes later have no idea who they are, what they look like.
>
> JAMES 1:22-24, THE MESSAGE

As we listen to our children, they will be mirrors to us of who we are and how we are doing in our journey as godly parents.

Feeding Your Baby

Scheduling your baby's feedings will probably be your first chance to apply your parenting style principles. You will read and hear extremes from "Don't have any schedule" to "Feed him every three hours, no matter what." Remember the models of the three parenting styles and see how you might apply these to how you will feed your baby.

The approach of feeding your baby on a strict schedule would fit the mentality of the parent-directed model. The parent is in control and decides what is best for the baby. What is best is predetermined rather than based on the uniqueness of the baby's size or needs. Those who promote a preset schedule are sold on the benefits of an orderly household, a well-rested parent, and a baby who sleeps through the night.

The permissive approach to parenting favors feeding the baby on demand. Sometimes offering the breast can become the easiest solution to every cry. Most lactation specialists promote feeding on demand as the way to promote a rich milk supply and adequate weight gain for the baby.

The third option starts building trust, as your baby senses you are interested in his needs. With this approach, you offer food in addition to other possible solutions. You don't automatically eliminate food as the solution because it isn't time, and you don't assume first that food is the answer without assessing your baby's needs. The parent in this system gradually and gently guides the baby into a schedule, but doesn't rigidly impose a predetermined system of feeding. In some ways the come-alongside style of parenting combines the demand feeding approach with the goal of moving the infant onto a schedule. This is a team effort; the parent is the coach.

Although predetermined scheduling and demand feeding both offer convincing benefits, I promote the third option, with its clear, well-defined boundaries and room for the individuality of the baby. The structure, which is important for babies, is based on learning your child's natural rhythm. With this system you guide and nudge the newborn into a schedule led by her body and expressions of hunger, while incorporating the need to teach her to fit into life's system of eating during the day and sleeping at night. The parent trains the child to get her nights and days in sync with the rest of the family, but gives her plenty of time and room for individual ways of making that adaptation.

During the first two weeks after the baby's arrival, I would recommend ignoring a schedule and letting the baby, not the clock, guide your decisions. It would be better to err on the side of feeding too often during the day rather than not frequently enough. I would recommend feeding at least every three hours, perhaps even more often. This is especially true if you are breastfeeding.

The American Academy of Pediatrics has taken a position on the feeding of babies and has identified signs of hunger that will be of great help as you learn to discern your baby's needs: "Newborns should be nursed whenever they show signs of hunger, such as increased alertness or activity, mouthing or rooting. Crying is a late indicator of hunger. Newborns should be nursed approximately eight to twelve times every twenty-four hours until satiety."[1]

The more frequently you nurse, the faster your milk will come in and the less you will have to deal with nipple soreness. Nipple soreness usually has to do with how the baby is latching on. If you position the baby in a straight horizontal line across your chest, under and at your breast, and hold his chin down to open his mouth wide, latching on will be much easier and less traumatic to your nipples. To get help with brestfeeding, call the International Lactation Consultant Association at 919-787-5181 or La Leche League International at 847-519-7730.

Dear God our Father,

You nurture us. You hear our cries and respond to our needs. You have promised that You will be with us and provide for us. Give us the same sense of care and passion for our infant's needs for food. There will be times when we may have difficulty knowing whether she is hungry or just tired. Help us to have a calmness in listening and responding so she will develop a deep trust in us and in You. In Christ's name, Amen.

Managing Sleep Patterns

Managing your baby's sleep pattern is as important and controversial as feeding him. I believe it is vital to establish sleep routines right from the beginning, but how you do that is the key factor. I am most comfortable with the Sears' attitude (*Nighttime Parenting*) and I incorporate Weissbluth's findings.[2] Helpful neutral resources are *Baby & Child Care*[3] and *Caring for Your Baby and Young Child*.[4]

Putting the baby to sleep. Going to sleep is a conditioned or learned response. Consequently, wherever you decide your baby will sleep and however you will put him to sleep, you *must be consistent* if you are going to establish predictable sleep habits. Varying where and how you put a baby to sleep will cause him confusion and delay sleep-learning.

Helping the baby learn to sleep at night. Getting a baby to sleep through the night, unfortunately, is often a measure of a "good baby" or a "good parent." Don't even pursue this project until your baby is at least four months old and more than sixteen pounds. Even then, take your time. In my view, you enhance night sleeping by:

- Practicing consistency. Establish a routine that is calming; use rocking, singing, reading, praying, listening to soft music, or bathing. Sleep the baby in the same place or with similar conditions each time. Holding a sleeping infant is wonderful, but put him in his sleep place after he is calmed. If he awakens when you put him down, continue to assist him by patting, offering a pacifier, providing soothing background sounds, or allow him a minute or two to settle himself.
- Increasing frequency of daytime feedings (breast milk or formula during infancy; other potein—cheese, cottage cheese, yogurt, soy, and pureed baby meats—six times per day when older).
- Keeping night feedings short, quiet, dark, and relaxed. Even keep your body and breathing sleeplike. Avoid diaper changes unless very wet or dirty.
- Provide an environment conducive to sleep; ensure freedom from interruptions, temperature control, and some lightness differentiation for day and night.
- Assessing and correcting reasons for baby's awakening. Keep a log of sleeping and awakening times compared with eating patterns, activities, and day and night time routines. Determine and remove all allergens from the baby's and breastfeeding mom's diet. I recommend the elimination of newly introduced foods and the ELISA blood test for determination of food allergies.

Read the February 1999 and the March 2000 issues of *Parenting* magazine for techniques for sleep promotion for baby and older.[5]

Pray these words written for you:

Dear Father,

You have instructed us as parents to train our children according to their uniqueness with Your command to "train up a child in the way he should go" (Psalm 22:6). Help us to be able to discern the ways of this new baby and guide him into good sleep patterns that will benefit both him and us. Give us that perfect balance of structure and flexibility. In Jesus' name, Amen.

Prayers and Scripture

Listen to Me Under My Words
Oh God,
I come to you now
as a child to my Mother,
    out of the cold which numbs
        into the warm who cares.
Listen to me inside,
    under my words
        where the shivering is,
    in the fears
        which freeze my living,
    in the angers
        which chafe my attending,
    in doubts
        which chill my hoping,
    In the events
        which shrivel my thanking,
    in the pretenses
        which soften my loving.

Listen to me, Lord,
    as a Mother,
        and hold me warm,
        and forgive me.
Soften my experiences
    into wisdom,
my pride
    into acceptance,
my longing
    into trust,
and soften me
    into love
        and to others
        and to you.[6]

The heavens tell of the glory of God.
  The skies display his marvelous craftsmanship.
Day after day they continue to speak;
  night after night they make him known.
They speak without a sound or a word;
  their voice is silent in the skies;
yet their message has gone out to all the earth,
  and their words to all the world.

PSALM 19:1-4, NLT

The Seventh Month: Becoming a Family

The beginning of the end of pregnancy and the beginning of a new life chapter—that's how to look at the seventh month. Growth and preparation for labor and delivery are the events of this month, for both mother and baby. This is the time to think about maintaining your intimacy as a couple, while planning how best to handle the needs of your newborn.

O Lord God, when you give to your servants to endeavor any great matter, grant us also to know that it is not the beginning, but the continuing of the same to the end, until it be thoroughly finished, which yield the true glory; through him who for the finishing of your work laid down his life, our Redeemer, Jesus Christ.

FRANCIS DRAKE[1]

The Growing Baby

With each day that passes, your baby's ability to thrive outside your body increases. Experts say that during this month, your baby would have an 85 percent chance of surviving if born prematurely, putting her within the limits of premature viability.[2] Of course, delivery now would not be ideal. Your baby would still need the medical support of an incubator to keep her warm, since she lacks enough body fat to perform that function. Artificial respiration would be necessary because of an inability to keep the lungs inflated. She would also need extra protection from infections because of her weak immune system. Yet, with today's technology your premature baby would have a good chance of doing fine long-term.

Your baby is starting to fill out with fat, which will eventually take away some of the wrinkled look as well as the reddish color. The fine, downy hair covering his body is disappearing. He is growing larger and filling his living space. His position in the uterus can now be determined, but it can still shift. The goal is a head-down position.

Although your baby's brain and liver functions are still underdeveloped, his brain is growing rapidly. He can now register information with all five senses and is more aware of and will react more quickly to stimuli. His response to Mom's voice is almost immediate. He can feel and respond to the Braxton-Hicks contractions, when the uterus tightens, though the amniotic fluid cushions him and keeps him from being hurt by the contractions. Vision is the least used and least developed sense while in the womb, yet your baby is now looking around when he has his eyes open. He can discriminate between various levels of light and darkness, but can't yet detect objects. This visual activity is preparation for seeing after birth.

As the baby is getting stronger, he is moving, flexing his limbs, and even making grasping motions with his hands. Your little one is likely to be most active when you are sleeping, and to be sleeping when you are rocking him with your movements during the day.

Changes in the Mother-to-Be

Excitement and concern both seem to flutter inside most expectant mothers as they realize they are nearing the end of the pregnancy and approaching the time when they can finally embrace their little one. You may find yourself eager for the end result but overwhelmed with the things you need to do before you get there.

To have concerns about the health and well-being of your baby is completely normal. Ultrasound and other testing that is possible during pregnancy today give some sense of reassurance that the baby is OK. Yet, there are still many unknowns that can cause worry. The trek the baby has to make from the safety of your womb to the outside world is not an easy one, for him or you. Yet with the prenatal care and medical resources to monitor and manage labor and delivery, the probability of having a completely normal baby has never been better. Even when complications do arise or a child is born with a health problem, treatment and correction are readily available and effective for most.

Our grandson, Matthew, born to John and Julene, had been at home for only twenty hours when Julene and I observed Matthew having a very small, almost unidentifiable seizure. Within hours, and after six more seizures, he was on medication and his seizures were under control. The next eight days in pediatric intensive care were frightening and traumatic, as procedures of diagnosis and monitoring him led to the conclusion that Matthew had suffered a mild stroke, an extremely rare event in newborns.

I would not share this story, for fear of adding to your worries, except that the ending is so positive. Matthew started walking at ten and a half months of age and is a bright, responsive, happy little guy with absolutely no residual evidence of having had a stroke. Yes, there were some losses. His life didn't start out as expected. Julene and John didn't get much time to enjoy the excitement of bringing their first baby home. But the evidence of God's presence in that situation and the skill of the medical team can only really be known by the three of us—John, Julene, and myself—who were there for eight days, watching over Matthew twenty-four hours a day.

> Give your entire attention to what God is doing right now, and don't get worked up about what may or may not happen tomorrow. God will help you deal with whatever hard things come up when the time comes.
>
> MATTHEW 6:34, THE MESSAGE

Pray for confidence in God's presence with you and your baby.

Dear Father God,

We have confidence in You. You have promised that You care for everything about us and that You will help us through any situation we might face. We don't know what will happen in the next days, weeks, or months, but we do know that You are with our baby and us. Take all our concerns and worries. Help us to focus on those aspects of preparing for safe labor and delivery that are in our control and to leave the rest to You. In Jesus' name, Amen.

Hopefully, your excitement is more consuming than your anxiety. There is the excitement of seeing your baby. There is the excitement of having that warm, snuggly baby to love and adore. There is the excitement of sharing one of the most intimate experiences of life. There is the excitement of your body being free of the burden of the weight of the baby, the enlarged uterus, and the extra blood volume. There is the excitement of preparing the baby's diapers, toys, clothing, and place to sleep. Everything is so new and tiny and soft. And there is the excitement of noticing the changes in your body, preparing you to bring this baby into the world.

O God,
In the crush of traffic, the push and shove of shopping,
  the surge in corridors of school, we often wonder if
  we are known by you, or by any one else.
In the isolation of apartments, the solitude of speeding
automobiles, the seclusion of [our homes],
we often wonder if we are remembered by you,
or by anyone else.

 Remind us anew, this day, O God, that you have the whole wide world in your hands.

 Assure us, once more, that you know us, each one by name and by need.

 Let us never feel forsaken, nor believe that multitudes are outside your providence.

 Here and now, with fresh courage and full assurance, we call you Father, and together pray to you.

David M. Currie[3]

Most of the physical changes you are experiencing during this trimester are preparing you for labor and delivery. When the uterus contracts and relaxes, your body is practicing for birthing.

Your breasts are also preparing for childbirth, and are starting to produce colostrum to provide nourishment for the baby. This is a sticky, watery substance that will provide your baby's first food if you breastfeed. Leaking colostrum from your breasts during these final months of pregnancy is common.

Caution about clumsiness becomes the motto from now until birth. Due to shifts in the baby's position and changes in your uterus in preparation for delivery, you are more likely to lose your balance and to have accidents. Be alert as you walk up and down stairs, consciously maintain your posture, and do not climb up on things. Avoid slippery surfaces and generally practice caution.

Discomforts and limitations during this time are part of pregnancy. Your abdomen may ache more as the uterus stretches. Shortness of breath is usually due to the baby crowding into your breathing space as she grows, and is not an indication of lack of oxygen. Possible oxygen deprivation to the baby is one of the reasons air travel is not usually recommended after the seventh month. Altitude changes can affect the baby at this stage, and cramped sitting over an extended period of time is also not great for your circulation, since your abdomen is already putting so much pressure on the blood flow to your lower body. Furthermore, it is not wise to be far away from your regular medical practitioner this late in your pregnancy.

You can expect your prenatal visits to increase in frequency to every two weeks as your doctor keeps a careful watch over you and the baby at this stage. Another reminder: make sure you are taking your prenatal vitamin-mineral supplement and consuming plenty of calcium. Because of the rapid hardening of the baby's bones at this time, your calcium needs will be the greatest during these next few weeks, and you will want to have the maximum energy benefit of your supplement as you go into labor and delivery.

> And the Lord will continually guide you,
> And satisfy your desire in scorched places,
> And give strength to your bones;
> And you will be like a watered garden,
> And like a spring of water whose waters do not fail.
>
> ISAIAH 58:11, NASB

Decisions of the Month

Determine Parenting Roles

There are a number of issues involved in decisions about parenting and family responsibilities. How will you handle finances and working outside the home? Calculate your anticipated income. What other commitments do each of you have that will take you away from the care of the baby? Be deliberate as you choose and set limits on these outside commitments. If this is your first child, you may have no sense of how much you will be able to accomplish with a new baby. The child's personality and patterns of sleeping and eating, as well as your interaction with your child, will affect your decision.

How much time will either or both of you be able to take after the baby is born before you go back to work? Allow yourselves some recovery time. The better the mother takes care of herself, the stronger her muscles will be for future babies. The quicker the father catches up on his sleep, the more available he will be to allow the mother to recover. Family bonding and adjustment will be easiest if you can both be totally free of all outside commitments for two weeks (or longer, if finances and your work situation allow that luxury), but one week is better than none.

What resources do you have to call on after the baby is born, and which of those would you like to use when? After the first child, you may want to plan the first five days to a week for just the three of you. If you've had a long labor and delivery, you might want someone to come in for the first twenty-four hours to let the two of you sleep; after that you can take over. Some families hire a baby nurse for the first two weeks and love it. Others have extended family come to help right away. This is a very personal decision. If you have multiple births or a complication, you will need help immediately and continuously.

Invite grandparents or other helpers according to your needs and relationships. If you can, give them a sense of your thinking ahead of time. They may need to make some adjustments in their lives in order to be there for you.

Will you have help after the initial adjustment period? Your financial situation and outside responsibilities will influence this decision. To be able to be the best possible parent for your child, you may need to sacrifice other expenditures and get help, rather than be stressed to your limit.

After Greg, our second child, was born, I was able to be home for six months with pay because I was on a twelve-month pay–nine-month-work university system. I had worked for eighteen months, or six quarters, without taking a quarter off, so after his birth I had two quarters available.

When it was time for me to go back to work, I needed child

care. With Cliff a graduate student and me supporting us, we would never have dreamed of being able to hire full-time help. Yet, to our amazement, we discovered that we could hire a full-time, live-in helper for less money per week than an hourly babysitter. What a gift! When I was home I was able to devote my full attention to Julene and Greg, yet know that they were well cared for when I was away and that nothing else was being neglected while I spent my time with them. Check all of your options before you close the door on a prospect you might think impossible.

What roles and responsibilities do each of you see yourself and the other assuming? Who will get up at night? If the mother is breastfeeding and the father can manage it with his work schedule, it is nice if he can get up, change the baby's diaper, and bring the baby to Mom for nursing. If the mom can rest during the day and Dad has long hours at work, that system may not be reasonable.

Who will be the primary caretaker of the child? What does this mean to each of you? How will each of you be involved with the child? Who will wash the clothes, make the beds, load and unload the dishwasher, cook the meals? Maybe you will do everything jointly. Maybe you will have certain days when each of you is responsible.

Clarifying expectations ahead of time reduces tension and avoids disappointments. With the clarification, there also must be flexibility. The art of parenting is anticipating, planning, and then adjusting to the actual circumstances that arise. The goal is for the two of you to remain coordinated in your plans, duties, and expectations.

Tasks, Hopes, and Dreams for the Month

Choosing Names

Throughout Scripture, the choosing of names has significant meaning. Luke 2:21 reads: "And when eight days were completed before His circumcision, His name was then called Jesus, the name given by the angel before He was conceived in the womb"(NASB).

Brainstorming together as a couple or a family about your baby's name can be fun. Name books offer an endless supply of options. You may prefer a certain style of name, whether traditional or more trendy. You may come with certain criteria for a name. You may want to choose a name that can be shortened to a nickname or one that can't be shortened. Think about possible nicknames that could be a problem. Also, put the initials of the proposed name together and make sure they don't spell an embarrassing or negative word. You may want names that are distinctly feminine or masculine, rather than unisex. Maybe you come from a tradition of using family names in some way. Look up the meaning of the names that interest you.

When your child is born, if the name doesn't seem to fit, you may reconsider some previous choices or start again. You have a day or two after birth to complete the birth certificate.

Choosing Names for Grandparents

Deciding what your baby will call his grandparents can be a special connecting task to do with your parents. If the baby will have more than one set of grandparents, choosing differing names of endearment for the different sets, though not a necessity, may help him be less confused about the identity of each of his grandparents. Your families may have traditions. Our family has always used Grandma and Grandpa, so that is who we are. Fortunately, our kids' in-laws were used to other terms, like Nana, Grandmom, Papa, and Grandad. You may have more nontraditional terms. Just make sure both you and the grandparents like the choices.

Prayers and Scriptures

Heavenly Father,

We thank you for the life of this child entrusted to our care. Help us to remember that we are all your children, and so to love and nurture him, that he may attain to that full stature intended for him in your eternal kingdom. Amen.[4]

Dear Lord,

You promised the children of Israel that if they followed Your commands You would bless them. "If you obey the commands of the Lord your God and walk in his ways, the Lord will establish you as his holy people as he solemnly promised to do. Then all the nations of the world will see that you are a people claimed by the Lord, and they will stand in awe of you" (Deuteronomy 28:9-10, NLT). Lord, may we earn our children's awe by our life of following Your way. May the name we choose for our baby reflect your love for him. Amen.

God, brilliant Lord,
    yours is a household name.
Nursing infants gurgle choruses about you;
    toddlers shout the songs
That drown out enemy talk,
    and silence atheist babble.

PSALM 8:1-2, THE MESSAGE

I don't mean to say that I have already achieved these things or that I have already reached perfection! But I keep working toward that day when I will finally be all that Christ Jesus saved me for and wants me to be. No, dear brothers and sisters, I am still not all I should be, but I am focusing all my energies on this one thing: forgetting the past and looking forward to what lies ahead, I strain to reach the end of the race and receive the prize.

PHILIPPIANS 3:12-14, NLT

The Eighth Month: Preparing and Training

Training is an appropriate theme for this month. As mentioned previously, the strength and endurance required for labor and delivery would be best prepared for with the same amount of discipline as the athlete applies in preparing for a marathon. The baby is certainly doing her best to prepare for the jolt of managing life's functions outside the warmth and safety of the womb.

The Growing Baby

All of the baby's major systems are working overtime, attempting to complete their development before the uterus stars contracting intensely and regularly enough to push her out into the world. She is flexing her muscles, blinking her eyes, swallowing the amniotic fluid, and using the muscles that she will need for breathing. Even her hiccups prepare her for this task. Just as last month she trained her senses to hear, taste, feel, smell, and begin to see, she is now exercising the skills she will need to thrive after birth. She is practicing coordination, thumb sucking for soothing, dreaming, and even the motions of crying.

Pray for patience, tenderness, and discernment in response to your baby's cries. Pray in your own words or use these written for you:

Dear Heavenly Father,

You have reassured us that when we cry to You, You hear us and You know our needs before we say them. Fill us with a sense of Your presence, and empower us with that ability to tenderly and patiently listen to our child and anticipate her needs. In Jesus' name, Amen.

Even though most babies born at this time will do well because the air sacs of the lungs are now lined with a liquid (a surfactant) that keeps them from collapsing, the growth and maturation of the last two months are extremely valuable. The immunities she is acquiring from the antibodies that pass through the placenta from your body will be an important protection for her after birth. Your baby will almost double her weight during this month alone. If she were born now, she still might need an incubator because she might not have enough fat yet to keep herself warm. As she nears the end of the month she might do just fine without assistance.

If your baby has not moved herself into the head-down position by the end of the seventh month, she probably will do so sometime this month. As she grows, she fills the uterine space and has more difficulty turning. Smaller babies continue to turn and move until late in the pregnancy.

Changes in the Mother-to-Be

The baby's vigorous movements, which may make your last months of pregnancy rather uncomfortable, are her practice for thriving outside your body. Her body may push against your internal organs, making breathing difficult or causing heartburn.

Backaches are a likely consequence of the increased size and weight of the baby, the placenta, the uterus, and the amniotic fluid. In addition to the strain on your back because of the increased load you are carrying, the ligaments and muscles supporting the small of your back also will relax and loosen in preparation for labor and delivery. An exercise routine designed to prepare your body for childbirth will help your back and train your body.

The pressure and size of the uterus causes other discomforts as well. Urination frequency increases as the bladder has less room to expand. Do not be tempted to lessen your liquid intake, however. Pressure on your bowels can contribute to constipation. Fluids, fruits, vegetables, and fibers are even more important during these last two months. Calcium, fats, and proteins are vital for the rapid maturation of your baby that will occur in these last weeks. Pressure on your veins can cause aching in the legs. Avoid being on your feet or sitting in one position for long periods of time. Sleep may be difficult. Remember to sleep on your left side as much as possible to improve your and the baby's circulation. Use pillows to support your abdomen and to take the pressure off your back.

Each woman carries her baby differently, depending on her structure and the baby's size and position. Sometimes the baby is high in the abdomen, while other times it is lower in the pelvis. The baby be be all out in front, so that you hardly look pregnant from the back, or she may be in a position that makes you look wide. How you are carrying your baby affects how you feel.

As you reach the end of this month and know the baby will now be able to survive outside the womb, you will notice yourself relaxing, at least about the issues of premature birth. Don't think you're unusual if you sort of wish the baby would come early. The waiting can seem endless. Yet, I would encourage you to relish these last days with your husband and any other children.

> Yet you do not know what your life will be like tomorrow. Be patient, therefore.... Behold the farmer waits for the precious produce of the soil, being patient about it, until it gets the early and late rains. You too be patient; strengthen your hearts.
>
> JAMES 4:14; 5:7, NASB

Say a prayer of praise to God for bringing you and your baby this far along.

O Lord, we have put our trust in You, and You have blessed us. You are our God! We are so thankful to have kept our baby in the womb this long, so that she has been able to reach a level of maturation where she could survive in the world, should she be born now. We pray that You will allow her birth to be timed at just the right moment for her. Protect her and us as we prepare for her arrival. Amen.

Decision of the Month

How Will You Handle the Baby's Crying?

Babies can't talk, so they communicate by crying. Each baby is unique in her style and tone of crying. Your baby's crying doesn't have to make you anxious, but don't ignore her cries. Respond as you would like to be responded to when you are talking to someone. Look your baby in the eyes. Make sweet sounds back to the baby in tones that empathize appropriately with her cries. Let's say you are in the kitchen and the baby is napping in her bassinet. You hear her start to cry. You might call, "I'm coming; I'll be right there!" Or if it doesn't seem like she should be waking up quite yet, you might wait a few minutes to see if she settles herself back to sleep.

The mechanism of infant crying explains the different cries. The Sears' put it this way: "The baby senses a need. The realization of this need reflexively triggers the sudden inspiration of air, followed by a forceful expiration. The expelled air passes the vocal cords, and the vibrating cords produce a sound we call a cry. It is a signal triggered by a need. Babies will use different signals for different needs. The more intense the need, the more forceful the signal. These are called cry prints and are unique to each baby."[1] They are designed to elicit a response.

Initially, you shouldn't expect to be able to discern the meaning of each cry. That understanding will evolve as you listen and respond. You might verbalize various options to the baby, like, "Do you need your diaper changed?" "Are you hungry already?" "Are you feeling overstimulated?" "Are you needing Daddy's big arms?" The baby will sense your care even if she doesn't understand your exact words.

Charting the baby's crying patterns can be helpful. You might keep a spiral-bound notepad on a table near where the baby sleeps. You will quickly begin to better understand your baby's cries and your responses to them.

An infant whose needs are consistently and quickly met in the first six months cries less and shows less negative behavior in the second part of the year. Infants escalate into intense crying in about two minutes. If you get to your child before she switches into intense need-signal, she will be easier to calm and her signals will be less urgent in the future. The longer she is ignored, the more intense her cry will get and the more quickly her level of intensity will escalate in future cries for help.

Fussing is different from crying. Babies can be allowed to fuss. When fussing or giving a signal of a momentary or passing discomfort, the baby will settle on her own or soothe herself within two minutes.

If you are new parents, you will find comfort in knowing what are normal crying patterns for newborns. According to Marc Weissbluth, M.D., director of the Sleep Disorders Center at Children's Memorial Hospital in Chicago, "the average newborn cries relatively little during the first week, picks up the tempo at two weeks of age, and may reach a peak of three hours or more of daily crying time at six to eight weeks. Mercifully, the crying usually subsides by the third month to a more bearable one hour per day."

What can you do when your baby cries? Realize that the baby's crying will cause stress in you. Use breathing techniques and prayer to calm yourself. Call upon others when you can't get yourself calmed. Rock your infant. Rocking at a steady, slow pace is usually the most soothing. Vertical rocking at the pace of about one knee bend per second has been shown to win out over all other rocking in calming crying babies.[2] To rock your baby vertically, hold her upright in your arms while you are standing, then do rhythmic knee bends. (This is also a great way for Mommy to get back in shape.) Carry or hold your baby. Research at Montreal Children's Hospital has found that babies who are carried for more than four hours a day cry and fuss only half as much as do those who are carried for fewer hours. Calm interaction with your baby will help both parents and baby. Barry Brazelton's *Touchpoints* is an excellent resource for learning how to respond to your baby's crying.

Pray for calmness and discernment in listening and responding to your baby's cries. Pray silently with or without words. Picture yourself listening and responding to your baby crying. Get a sense of God's peace through the Holy Spirit filling you with deep love, care, and calm in response to your baby.

Dear Father,

Thank You for hearing my cries. Wrap Your arms around me. Give me a deep sense of peace in knowing that I my not be able to stop my baby's crying, just as You don't always take away my pain and struggles. Help me remember that You have promised that You will always be with me and will never desert me. As I put my trust in You, give me the calmness and consistent presence for my baby that You have granted me. In Jesus' name, Amen.

You will keep in perfect peace all who trust in You, whose thoughts are fixed on You!

ISAIAH 26:3, NLT

Tasks, Hopes, and Dreams for the Month

Enjoy Some Special Time

Life will change when the new baby arrives. Savor these last days for the two of you and with the rest of the children. Older children will adjust so much better if they feel securely loved and have been lavished with attention before the baby comes. Keep a balance between including them in the process of preparing for the baby and focusing on them without mention of the baby.

Have a Talk in Preparation for the Baby's Arrival

If your children are old enough, let them talk about their excitement and their concerns. Listen, reflect to ensure that you understand, and then validate their feelings. Also provide accurate information, to dispel worries. If children have differing feelings about the new baby, let them know that each of their reactions is normal and that it is just fine for people to react differently when facing changes in life. You as a couple may have differences as well. You may want to share examples of these differences that will not make children anxious.

For a young child who can't identify and verbalize feelings as easily, this would be a great time to buy a playhouse with rooms and little people. Set up the rooms in a manner similar to how your home is set up now, with figures representing Mom, Dad, and other children. Let the child move the toy people around to portray a day at home. Sometime before he loses interest, pretend Daddy is at work and have him come home to take Mommy to the hospital, or act out your specific plans for the beginning of labor. Continue the play, dropping the children off at their friends' houses or having a caretaker come into the playhouse before Mommy and Daddy leave. Once Mommy has the baby, have the children come to a play hospital to see the baby, if that is allowed where you will be delivering (you can make the hospital room with a small box, using cloth or tissues for beds.)

Then have all of you arrive home with the baby. Have your child talk for the play child. Continue as long as your child is interested.

Not all of this play preparation has to be done this month or at one time. The younger the child, the longer you will need to wait and the less information you will be able to give at one time. Let the child lead you in this with his ability to participate and attend.

Choosing a Pediatrician

The process of choosing your baby's doctor is similar to the process you used in choosing your own practitioner. The person who cares for your baby must be someone you trust and can relate to comfortably. These two qualities aren't always apparent in one professional. Some physicians have great interpersonal skills, but not as strong a medical reputation. Others lack bed side manner but would be the one you would want to determine and manage your child's medical treatment in case of serious illness, surgery, or injury. Your goal is to find a professional who embodies both of these important qualities.

To find the ideal pediatrician for you, talk to friends who have babies and to personnel at the hospital you would hope to use if the need arose. Get a list of recommendations with pros and cons from your maternity care specialist and ask questions that are important for you.

Once you have interviewed several possible pediatricians, their differences, along with your gut reaction to the appearance of the office, the staff (often you will be talking with the staff rather than the physician), and the responses to your questions, will inform your decision. Remember to follow up all physician interviews with a courtesy call regarding your decision.

Dear God,

Open our eyes. Give us a sense of discernment. Lead us to the professional who will be just the right person for our baby and our family. We trust your guidance. Amen.

Prayers and Scripture

God, the one and only—
    I'll wait as long as he says.
Everything I hope for comes from him,
    So why not?
He's solid rock under my feet,
    Breathing room for my soul,
An impregnable castle:
    I'm set for life.

                    PSALM 62:5-6, THE MESSAGE

Give me, O Lord, a steadfast heart, which no unworthy affection may drag downwards; give me an unconquered heart, which no tribulation can wear out; give me an upright heart, which no unworthy purpose may tempt aside. Bestow on me also, O Lord my God, understanding to know you, diligence to seek you, wisdom to find you, and a faithfulness that may finally embrace you, through Jesus Christ our Lord. Amen

Thomas Aquinas[3]

Birth, like love, is energy and a process. Both unfold with their own timing, with a uniqueness that can never be anticipated, with a power that can never be controlled, but with an exquisite mystery to be appreciated.[1]

The Ninth Month: Nearing the End

You're on your final lap, and so am I! There is an amazing similarity between pregnancy and writing a book. Authors and mothers both often pass their due dates. The processes of bringing a baby into the world and sending a book to press take focus, hard work, and dedication, but the products are well worth the effort. Neither is ever perfect, but both evoke pride in their producers.

> This is what the Lord says: Do not be afraid! Don't be discouraged.... stand still and watch the Lord's victory. He is with you.... Do not be afraid or discouraged. Go out there tomorrow, for the Lord is with you!
>
> 2 CHRONICLES 20:15b,17b, NLT

The Growing Baby

Your baby's growth is awesome, especially that of his brain. His head circumference continues to increase during this month to accommodate this critical brain development period. His little body may actually be getting chubby as fat deposits are being added day by day. Full baby cheeks are the result of these fat deposits and the powerful sucking muscles that have developed, probably from thumb sucking while in the womb. During the last ten days of gestation, or from day 265 on, the baby will gain half an ounce every day that he stays in the uterus. The change of cartilage to bone has been a steady process in the baby that will not be complete at birth. You can be happy about that fact because cartilage is flexible and easier to move through the birth canal than solid bone.

During the last few months, your baby will have acquired from you an immunity to any diseases you have had or have been immunized against. He will continue to receive these disease-combating antibodies from you until birth. After birth he will receive protection through your breast milk if you choose to breastfeed.

The baby has reached his size limit by the end of this month, and you have probably reached the limit of your ability to hold any more of him, so his growth will slow while you wait for his signal system to set labor into motion. He is now physically mature and ready to be born.

Everything God created is good, and to be received with thanks. Nothing is to be sneered at and thrown out. God's Word and our prayers make every item in creation holy.

1 TIMOTHY 4:4-5, THE MESSAGE

Say a silent prayer of praise and protection for your baby. Praise God for His creation of your child, and picture God's protection surrounding your baby now, during birth, and throughout life.

Changes in the Mother-to-Be

As your baby becomes cramped and his movement gets restricted, you will feel the tightness and fullness of his increased size. Clumsiness, shortness of breath, leg cramps, swollen ankles, and urinary frequency are discomforts you'll have to live with for a while longer. Relief of pressure on your respiratory and digestive systems will be welcome when the baby drops and engages in the pelvis. This drop is called "settling" or "lightening." Unfortunately, pressure on your bladder and legs will increase at this time. Take time to get off your feet, but also continue your exercises. Walking is great preparation for labor and delivery, even through the early stages of labor.

Pray a prayer of petition as you use these words or your own to express your needs at this time:

Dear God,

During this final month, bless me with an extra dose of patience, comfort, and strength. Help me have a keen sense of judgment as I attempt to match my available energy with the demands on my time. Keep my focus on You, and may I continually experience Your presence with my family and me. I give myself to You. Make my life complete. Amen.

Yahweh made my life complete
    when I placed all the pieces before him.

When I got my act together,
    he gave me a fresh start.
Now I'm alert to God's ways;
    I don't take God for granted.
Every day I review the ways he works;
    I try not to miss a trick.
I feel put back together,
    and I'm watching my step.
Yahweh rewrote the text of my life
    when I opened the book of my heart to his eyes.

PSALM 18:20-24, THE MESSAGE

Your body is gearing up for the birth of your baby. Your energy level will fluctuate more during this month than it has at any other time during the pregnancy. Moments of fatigue will alternate with great spurts of energy. Use those energetic times wisely. At the same time that you need all the rest you can get, the baby may be awakening you at night, and you may be thinking about all the tasks you "need" to accomplish before he arrives. I always reminded myself that when babies come early their mothers seem to manage without having completed their "to-do" lists. You might differentiate between tasks that would be difficult for someone else to complete and are critical for a successful transition into parenting this new baby and those that would be great to have finished before the baby comes but won't impact life if they don't get done.

Your practitioner will want to see you every week from now until the baby comes. These appointments are important to monitor changes and check any problems immediately. Prelabor contractions increase at this time, and the doctor will monitor their intensity and frequency. Internal exams will now be part of your weekly visits. Write down instructions from your practitioner and questions you want to remember to ask. Even though these instructions and thoughts seem clear at first, they may become blurry or be forgotten later. Remember, you are juggling many feelings, thoughts, and preparations.

Because your body is preparing itself for blood loss during delivery, your blood volume is rapidly increasing. The increase in your internal blood volume can add a couple of pounds of weight. This blood volume weight gain may not be evidenced on the scale, however, because this month might also be accompanied by the loss of a few pounds due to your increased metabolism, designed to supply the extra energy demands of the baby.

Dear Father,

Thank You for Your promises to supply all of our needs. Give my body what it requires to be able to supply my baby's needs during this last spurt of growth before birth. Fill me, dear Lord, with the capacity to give far beyond my human ability. In Jesus' name, Amen.

Maintain your fluid intake and good eating habits. Your iron intake is critical during this month, both for you and for the baby. The baby is storing iron to maintain his iron supplies for the first four months after birth. Even if you can't eat as much because there isn't room for your stomach to expand, eat healthily and frequently. You need the energy.

I love Thee, O Lord, my strength.
The Lord is my rock and my fortress and my deliverer,
My God, my rock, in whom I take refuge;
My shield and the horn of my salvation, my stronghold.
I call upon the Lord, who is worthy to be praised....

Make me know Thy ways, O Lord;
Teach me Thy paths.
Lead me in Thy truth and teach me,
For Thou art the God of my salvation;
For Thee I wait all the day.
Remember, O Lord, Thy compassion
   and Thy lovingkindnesses.

PSALM 18:1-3; 25:4-6, NASB

Decision of the Month

Dealing With Pain During Labor

Your decision about pain management will depend somewhat on the physical preparation you have been doing and will continue to do until the time of labor and delivery. It will also depend on your pain threshold and on your practitioner's opinion. Don't hesitate to ask about anything that concerns you. The more you know, the better you will feel about your final choices.

Allow your pain management decision to be flexible. You might have several optional plans, depending on how the labor progresses. For example, if your baby is posterior, your labor is likely to be longer and felt in the back (referred to as back labor). In this case it will feel as if the baby is trying to get out but is pressing against your tailbone rather than your vagina. Her pushing will likely be painful to your back but will not dilate your cervix. The practitioner may try to turn the baby during labor. You may be encouraged to get on your hands and knees to help the baby turn by herself.

Having thought through your choices and the pros and cons

of the various options for pain management will be a huge benefit when you are actually in the situation of needing help to bring this baby into the world. Work with your body. Don't fight the pain; rather move toward it and breathe with it. Ask for pain medication when that will make the process more productive for you. Trust yourself to know what you need, even as you rely on your husband or coach and your practitioner.

Tasks, Hopes, and Dreams for the Month

Prepare for Labor
- Keep emergency phone numbers handy.
- A bloody show or extra mucus is usually a sign that the mucus plug sealing the opening of the uterus has dislodged, and you may go into labor within hours or days.
- Bright red discharge or persistent spotting should be reported to the doctor.
- If your water breaks, notify your practitioner immediately.
- Contractions that begin in your lower back, increasing in pain and intensity, spreading to your lower abdomen, and building in a wave that cannot be interrupted by change in position must be timed and reported. Measure both the length of the contraction and the time between the start of one and the start of the next.
- Diarrhea with a contraction may be a sign of labor.

Become even more diligent in setting aside time for the recommended exercises, especially breathing, relaxation, and preparation for labor and delivery exercises.

Make Preparations to Ease Stress After the Baby's Birth

Arrange for as much help as you can afford or is offered to you without setting up too much commotion in your household. Prepare food to freeze. If friends ask how they can help, schedule dinners to arrive every other evening for the first week or two. When people bring food as a gift, they often bring far too much for one meal, which is great for leftovers. If you are breastfeeding, let them know ahead of time that it would be best if you avoided garlicky, spicy, or gaseous foods. Stock up on the best frozen vegetables, so you can get a sufficient supply without frequent visits to the market for fresh produce.

Prepare Your Bags for the Hospital

Baby's bag. The baby won't need much. The hospital will provide diapers, but you will want to bring an outfit and a blanket in which to bring her home. You will need to have an approved infant car seat before you can take the baby home in the car. In addition, you might want to prepare her diaper bag with the supplies basic to a baby's care, so that it is always ready to go.

Your bag. This might include:
- a stop clock or watch for timing contractions
- any supplies you have used for relaxation or preparation
- camera or equipment to record this life event
- personal cosmetics and body care items
- lip balm and sugarless lollipops to keep your lips moist
- lots of bottled drinking water
- high energy snacks that are soothing and easy to digest
- comfortable sleepwear
- a robe that opens down the front if you plan to breastfeed
- maternity or nursing bras and pads (several)
- panties and extra absorbent and thick sanitary pads

- an outfit to go home in that opens down the front and is oversized and loose, such as an early maternity outfit
- a breast pump

Prayers and Scripture

Trust in the Lord with all your heart; do not depend on your own understanding. Seek his will in all you do, and he will direct your paths.

Don't be impressed with your own wisdom. Instead, fear the Lord....

Happy is the person who finds wisdom and gains understanding.... Wisdom is a tree of life to those who embrace her; happy are those who hold her tightly.

My child, don't lose sight of good planning and insight. Hang on to them, for they fill you with life and bring you honor and respect. They keep you safe on your way and keep your feet from stumbling.

PROVERBS 3:5-7, 13, 18, 21-23, NLT

O Lord, our Lord, the majesty of your name fills the earth! Your glory is higher than the heavens. You have taught children and nursing infants to give you praise.... When I look at the night sky and see the work of your fingers—the moon and the stars you have set in place—what are mortals that you should think of us, mere humans that you should care for us? For you made us only a little lower than God, and you crowned us with glory and honor. You put us in charge of everything you made, giving us authority over all things.... O Lord, our Lord, the majesty of your name fills the earth!

PSALM 8:1-9, NLT

ﬁnd Joseph also went up from Galilee ... to the city of David ... in order to register, along with Mary, who was engaged to him, and was with child. And it came about that while they were there, the days were completed for her to give birth. And she gave birth to her first-born son.

LUKE 2:4-7, NASB

The Time Is Here!

It's birth time. You have reached your due date. Only 5 percent of mothers (one in twenty) deliver on their due date,[1] partly because the calculation of that date is an estimate from the last menstrual period rather than from an actual conception date. First-time mothers most often deliver after their due date.

There is a time for everything, a season for every activity under heaven. A time to be born.... God has made everything beautiful for its own time. And I know that whatever God does is final. Nothing can be added to it or taken from it.

ECCLESIASTES 3:1-2, 11, 14, NLT

Say a prayer of praise for your full-term pregnancy.

Dear God,

How wonderful You are. You have been our strength. You have blessed us with patience and trust in You. You have been with us to the end. We claim Your promise: "He gives childless couples a family, gives them joy as the parents of children. Hallelujah!" (Psalm 113:9, THE MESSAGE). Amen.

Labor, the process by which the baby passes from the uterus through the birth canal to the outside world, is actually initiated by the baby. She releases a hormone that makes the uterus start contracting with a different intensity, persistence, and regularity than in all previous contractions. It's as though she says, "Ready or not, here I come."

Say a prayer for protection for you and the baby: Picture the baby pushing against the cervix of your uterus. Picture yourself working with your baby to ease her journey. Picture God's strength filling you. Pray these words written for you:

Dear God,

You are our strength. You have designed my body to bear this baby. You have designed our precious baby. Protect her, dear Lord. We ask with intense passion for Your mercy, Your care, and Your presence and blessing during these hours of labor and delivery. Our trust is in You! Amen.

Labor is divided into three stages. The first stage starts with the first true contraction and ends when your cervix is fully dilated and effaced. That is a long process for most first-time moms. The second stage starts at full dilation and ends when the baby is pushed out of the vagina. The third stage starts after the birth and ends with the delivery of the placenta. You aren't likely to pay much attention to that part. You will be focused on your baby.

To give you some sense of what to expect, the first stage is best divided into three phases.[2] *The latent phase* lasts about six to eighteen hours for first-time moms, but may go on for as long as twenty hours. In subsequent labors, this first phase will last from two to ten hours. You may be able to remain active during the first hours. The more you walk and squat, the more pressure will be put on the cervix by the force of gravity, which will help your labor progress and keep your muscles from tensing. The contractions of the latent stage thin (or efface) the cervix so it can open (or dilate) to let the baby out. The cervix is like a thick, tight turtleneck on a sweater that you first roll down—that's the effacing—and then hold open—that's the dilating—to get your head through it.

During *the active phase,* most of the dilation takes place. Relaxation and breathing exercises with coaching will help you work with the contractions rather than against them. The uterus, with its concentrated efforts, is now accomplishing more in less time. Contractions are two to three minutes apart and more intense, opening the cervix to about eight centimeters.

From the end of the active phase through the third phase, *the transition phase,* you will need all the support and coaching you can get. This is the time an epidural or other medical pain management may be helpful. There will be little break time between contractions. When you reach full dilation of ten centimeters, the second stage of labor will begin.

Gracious and holy Father, give me wisdom to perceive you, intelligence to fathom you, patience to wait for you, eyes to behold you, a heart to meditate upon you, and a life to proclaim you, through the power of the Spirit of Jesus Christ our Lord.

Benedict[3]

Pray a prayer for those assisting you.

Dear Father,

I ask for patience and for stamina for my husband. Dear God, give him just the right words of encouragement at my time of need. I pray also for everyone who will care for me and our baby. Be present in the room. Give quickness of mind and alert decision-making. We depend on You, O Lord. In Your name, Amen.

The second stage of labor lasts about thirty minutes to three hours for first-time moms and five to thirty minutes for subsequent pregnancies. You will work with your contractions now to push the baby through the birth canal. The breathing exercises and your previous preparation for childbirth will give both parents confidence and skill in handling this stage of the birth process.

I Need to Breathe Deeply
Eternal Friend,
Grant me ease
To breathe deeply of this moment,
    this miracle now.
Precious Lord,
Grant me
    a sense of humor
        that adds perspective to compassion,
    gratitude
        that adds persistence to courage,

quietness of spirit
   that adds irrepressibility to hope,
openness of mind
   that adds surprise to joy,
That with gladness of heart
I may link arm and arm
With the One who opens my eyes and my ears
   To savor this moment
      Of grace and joy.[4]

Pray for strength in these words written by the psalmist:

The Lord is my Shepherd; I have everything I need. He lets me rest in green meadows; he leads me beside peaceful streams. He renews my strength. He guides me along right paths, bringing honor to his name. Even though I walk through the dark valley I will not be afraid, for you are close beside me. Your rod and your staff protect and comfort me. My cup overflows with blessings.

PSALM 23:1-5, NLT

There is an indescribable release of emotions when your baby is born. The third stage of labor lasts five to ten minutes and requires little of the mother. The person delivering the baby may ask you to give one last push to help the placenta separate from the wall of the uterus and descend down the vagina.

Care of the baby and evaluation of his condition follow delivery, either before or after you put your baby to the breast. You will need to be monitored while you recover. Once you are reunited, this is a wonderful time for your new family.

Pray this ready-made prayer for your newborn baby:

Lord, how I praise you for this new life you've entrusted to me. My child is fearfully and wonderfully made. Children are a reward from you, so I thank you for this blessing. Help me to wisely nurture my child. May this dear baby grow in wisdom and stature and favor with God and man, as Jesus did. Please protect and direct his/her steps, and may my child's life bring honor and glory to you. Amen.[5]

O Lord, our Lord, the majesty of your name fills the earth! Your glory is higher than the heavens. You have taught children and nursing infants to give you praise.

PSALM 8:1-2, NLT

In prayer we establish our personal relationship with God. The process of communicating with God through prayer has to be learned. You may have had years of comfortable interaction with God, or you may feel awkward in expressing your concerns and joys to God, your Father. Hopefully through these nine months, this book's guidance of your prayers regarding your baby and your pregnancy will have given you ways to articulate your feelings. You can rely on the Holy Spirit, who lives in you, to help you and teach you how to pray if expressing yourself to God does not come easily. Prayer brings us into the presence of God and requires that we listen as well as speak. We are humbled through prayer as we recognize that without God we can do nothing.

Dr. Billy Graham, in his book *Peace With God,* compares our communication with God to a baby's interaction with his parents: "Prayer is communicating. A baby's first response is to his parents. He isn't asking for anything. He is simply smiling back when his parents smile, cooing when they talk to him. What a thrill his response brings to the entire family! In the same way can you imagine the joy our first response to Him brings to God?"[6]

> Since ... we have confidence to enter the holy place by the blood of Jesus ... let us draw near with a sincere heart in full assurance of faith.
>
> HEBREWS 10:19, 22, NASB

Enter your relationship with this new baby with great confidence and joy as you walk arm in arm with the Giver of all love, strength, confidence, and wisdom. Trust in the Lord for every decision and acknowledge Him, and He will direct your steps along the wonderful road of parenting.

Blessings!

NOTES

On Prayer

1. C.S. Lewis, *Letters To Malcolm: Chiefly on Prayer* (New York: Harvest/ABJ Book, Harcourt, Brace Jovanovich, 1964), 9–13.
2. Lewis, 16–17.

On Pregnancy

1. Louise Bachelder, ed., *To Mother* (White Plains, N.Y.: Peter Pauper, 1971), 34.
2. Neil Clark Warren, *Living With the Love of Your Life and Loving It* (Colorado Springs: Focus on the Family, 1999).
3. Harville Hendrix, *Getting the Love You Want* (San Francisco: Harper & Row, 1990).
4. Tracie Hotchner, *Pregnancy and Childbirth* (New York: Avon, 1990), 55.
5. "Where Health Begins," *Newsweek*, September 27, 1999, 50–57.
6. M. Edward Davis, M.D., and Reva Rubin, *Obstetrics for Nurses* (Philadelphia: W.B. Saunders, 1962), 113–15.
7. Hotchner, 58.
8. To calm your concerns, refer to *Peace of Mind During Pregnancy,* by Christine Kelly-Bouchanan and *Will It Hurt the Baby? The Safety of Medications During Pregnancy and Breastfeeding,* by Richard S. Abrams, M.D.
9. Adapted from Bridget Swinney, "Whole 9 Months," *Parenting*, May 1999, 47.
10. Clifford L. Penner and Joyce J. Penner, *Men and Sex* (Nashville, Tenn.: Nelson, 1997).
11. Clifford Penner and Joyce Penner, *Sex Facts for the Family* (Waco, Tex.: Word, 1992), 88–93.

On Parenting

1. "Commitment to Excellence," International Congress on Christian Counseling, Atlanta, Ga. 1988, C2.
2. From *Toward Jerusalem* by Amy Carmichael, copyright The Dohnavur Fellowship 1936, published by Christian Literature Crusade. Used by permission.

3. M. Scott Peck, *The Road Less Traveled* (New York: Simon & Schuster, 1998).

4. Some great resources for positive parenting are *The Key to Your Child's Heart*, by Gary Smalley; *How to Talk So Kids Will Listen and Listen So Kids Will Talk*, by Faber and Mazlish; *Power of Parents' Words*, by H. Norman Wright; *Child Behavior*, by Ilg, Ames, and Baker; *Parenting Isn't for Cowards*, by Dr. James Dobson; and *How to Give Your Child a Great Self-Image*, by Dr. Debra Phillips.

5. Beth Wilson Saavedra, *Meditations for New Mothers* (New York: Workman, 1992), 244.

6. Daniel Partner, ed., *The One-Year Book of Personal Prayer* (Wheaton, Ill.: Tyndale, 1991), January 5.

7. Robin Currie, *Baby Bible Storybook* (Colorado Springs: Chariot Victor, 1994).

8. Georgie Adams, *The Bible Storybook* (New York: Dial, 1995).

9. Cyndy Szekeres, *A Small Child's Book of Prayers* (New York: Scholastic, 1999).

10. Dr. Marion Durfee, medical director, Pasadena Child Guidance Clinic.

The First Month

1. Adapted from Quin Sherrer and Ruthanne Garlock, *Prayers Women Pray* (Ann Arbor, Mich.: Servant, 1998), 27.

2. David Bodanis, *The Body Book* (Boston: Little, Brown and Company, 1984), 131.

3. Adele Faber and Elaine Mazlish, *Siblings Without Rivalry* (New York: Avon, 1987), 35–36.

4. Sherrer and Garlock, 91.

The Second Month

1. Partner, February 14.

2. David E. Rosage, *Follow Me: A Pocket Guide to Daily Scriptural Prayer* (Ann Arbor, Mich.: Servant, 1982), 59.

3. To check the safety of medications, look them up in a *Physicians' Desk Reference,* available at your local library or your pharmacy. Also see note 8 in "On Pregnancy" for two helpful resources.

4. *The Book of Common Prayer* (New York: Oxford University Press, 1990), 138.

The Third Month

1. Bodanis, 143.
2. Partner, February 10.
3. Sherrer and Garlock, 42.

The Fourth Month

1. Kim Boyce, *Dreams I'm Dreaming* (Ann Arbor, Mich.: Servant, 1997), 72.
2. Hotchner, 527.
3. Julene Stellato, child and adolescent psychologist, Rush Presbyterian Hospital, Chicago, interview, September 20, 1999.
4. Jane MacDougall, ed., *Pregnancy Week-by-Week* (London: Carol & Brown, 1997), 51.

The Sixth Month

1. Joe M. Sanders Jr., M.D., *AAP NEWS,* American Academy of Pediatrics, May 1998.
2. Marc Weissbluth, M.D., *Healthy Sleep Habits, Happy Child* (New York: Fawcett, 1999).
3. Paul C. Reisser, M.D., *Baby & Child Care* (Wheaton, Ill.: Tyndale, 1997).
4. Steven P. Shelov, M.D., ed., *Caring for Your Baby and Young Child* (New York: American Academy of Pediatrics, Bantam, 1994).
5. Christina Frank, "Sleep Through the Night," *Parenting,* February 1999, 87–91; Pamela Martin, "Sleep-well Strategies for Babies on Up," *Parenting,* March 2000, 98–104.
6. Ted Loder, *Guerrillas of Grace* (San Diego: LuraMedia, 1984), 16.

The Seventh Month

1. Partner, January 26.
2. MacDougall, 51
3. Partner, February 23. Reproduced from *Come, Let Us Worship God: A Handbook of Prayer for Leaders of Worship,* by David M. Currie. © 1977 The Westminster Press. Used by permission of John Knox Press.
4. *The Book of Common Prayer,* 841.

The Eighth Month

1. William Sears and Martha Sears, *Parenting the Fussy Baby and High Need Child* (New York: Little & Brown, 1996), 32.
2. Stellato.
3. Partner, January 5.

The Ninth Month

1. Gayle Peterson, *Birthing Normally* (Berkeley, Calif.: Shadow & Light, 1991).

The Time Is Here!

1. Lars Hamberger, *As Your Baby Grows From Conception to Birth* (New York: K-III Magazine Corporation, 1996), 14.
2. A great resource for labor and delivery is the chapter "Labor and Delivery" in *What to Expect When You Are Expecting* by Arlene Eisenberg, Heidi E. Murkoff, and Sandee E. Hathaway (New York: Workman, 1991).
3. Partner, February 19.
4. Adapted from Loder, 22–23.
5. Sherrer and Garlock, 43.
6. Billy Graham, *Peace With God* (Minneapolis: World Wide Publications, 1953), 169.